Praise for *Dr. Kellyann's Cleanse and Reset*

"If you are feeling tired, unhealthy, and emotionally burned out and want a fresh way to rejuvenate, Kellyann has a message for you: she's been where you are. And she knows the way out."

—Mehmet Oz, MD

"Dr. Kellyann proves that a cleanse doesn't need to be harsh to work. This painless plan, centered around delicious foods packed with healing nutrition, gives you big results without stress or starvation."

—Mark Hyman, MD, #1 *New York Times* bestselling author of *Food: What the Heck Should I Eat*

"This cleanse gets the job done fast—and the hearty soups, rich shakes, and refreshing green drinks will keep you satisfied from start to finish."

—JJ Virgin, *New York Times* bestselling author of *The Virgin Diet* and *The Sugar Impact Diet*

"The most profound discovery I made on my own journey to wellness was the healing power of food—a power that Dr. Kellyann harnesses in this brilliant plan."

—Dr. Izabella Wentz, #1 *New York Times* bestselling author of *Hashimoto's Thyroiditis* and *Hashimoto's Protocol*

"I absolutely love this cleanse—it's so easy and gentle, and it takes off extra pounds fast. If you're looking for a cleanse that restores and invigorates you, this is it."

—Penelope Ann Miller, award-winning stage, film, and TV actress

"I'm a huge fan of collagen, and I love cleanses—and Dr. Kellyann's plan combines the best of both worlds. Try it, and get more beautiful inside and out."

—Elena George, eight-time Emmy Award–winning celebrity makeup artist

"Do your body a big favor and try this quick, easy, science-based cleanse. You're going to love the results."

—Am and wellness expert

Dr. Kellyann's
Cleanse
and *Reset*

Detoxify, Nourish, and Restore Your Body for
Sustained Weight Loss . . . in Just 5 Days

Kellyann Petrucci, MS, ND

RODALE

New York

Copyright © 2019 by Best of Organic, LLC

All rights reserved.
Published in the United States by Rodale Books, an imprint of Random House, a division of Penguin Random House LLC, New York.
rodalebooks.com

RODALE and the Plant colophon are registered trademarks of Penguin Random House LLC.

Originally published in hardcover in the United States by Rodale, an imprint of the Crown Publishing Group, a division of Penguin Random House LLC, New York, in 2019.

Library of Congress Cataloging-in-Publication Data
LCCN number: 2019009988

ISBN 978-1-9848-2684-8
Ebook ISBN 978-1-9848-2668-8

Printed in the United States of America

Book design by Nicole LaRoche
Cover design by Jessie Sayward Bright
Cover photograph by Keith Major

10 9 8 7 6 5 4 3 2 1

First Paperback Edition

To Dr. Mehmet Oz and his team:
Brilliant, innovative, and passionate about delivering the truth.
Thank you for believing in me, elevating me so graciously,
and making me part of your Dr. Oz family.

Contents

Foreword

I have listened to, supported, laughed with, and cried with many people—mostly women in the dressing rooms of my stores. I am a fashion retailer, and I've been on the sales floor since I was fourteen years old, selling shoes in my family business in New York. Later, my family and I moved to California, where I started elysewalker in 1999. I am known as a "fashionista," but the truth is I am a mother, wife, girlfriend, and tomboy (mum's the word).

I have struggled with my weight and body image for as long as I can remember. I am not heavy, but I am not skinny. I am naturally a "medium." And I know I'm not alone in this struggle because I work with women, and now men, every day of the year, dressing them, styling them, and listening to their stories. Whether it's hormones, pregnancy, divorce, cancer, menopause, autoimmune disease, wedding celebrations, or bar mitzvahs, I get a little slice of all of my clients' lives.

At thirty-five, I was diagnosed with an autoimmune disease that attacks the irises of my eyes. (Remember, the definition of an autoimmune disease is your body wrongfully attacks healthy cells.) For about three years I struggled with daylight and overall light sensitivity, which led to steroids, weight gain, and then methotrexate to help get my body out of attack mode.

By forty I was doing great, searching for ways to create a healthy lifestyle and keep my body in remission. I read every book I could get my hands on and met with more than twenty-eight doctors over the years. I was gluten-free and I had everything under control: weight, eyes, exercise, and work-life balance.

Then, toward the end of my forties, my hormones started slowing down and all my usual tricks were no longer working for me. I felt exhausted and bloated (like five months' pregnant). My skin and hair started changing, and not in a good way. While my body was thickening, my hair was thinning. Not a good combo!

I am usually the caregiver and confidante, and I try to be a good role model for everyone on my team, both at work and in my private life. But now I needed help and support. My dad's wife, Lynn, and then my dear friend from Columbia University, Rebecca, and her husband, Peter, recognized my struggle and kept pushing me to read *Dr Kellyann's Bone Broth Diet*. I quickly told them, "Don't worry, I've got this. I'm gluten-free, I exercise, I will figure this out." But I didn't. And my struggle grew and grew as my old ways no longer delivered any results. So I read the book.

Once in a while, we all receive gifts. Dr. Kellyann has been a gift given to me by my friends and family. I read her book and started the diet with a group of friends (thank you, Michelle, Michael, Kath, and Deb). Together we built a team and checked in with one another daily. We started having dinner parties, bone broth–style, using Dr. Kellyann's delicious recipes. I couldn't believe it! My body was responding! I reached out to Dr. Kellyann personally and said I was going to be in New York, and would she like to join me for the Jonathan Simkhai fashion show? We met waiting in line at Spring Studios in Tribeca. She was wearing super-chic winter white, head to toe. And I knew I was going to love her!

Smart, bold, warm, funny, and totally approachable, Dr. Kellyann has become my spiritual gangster. She is Italian and will tell you, "Hey, I love to eat!" My kind of girl! She understands the inflammation that so many of us struggle with. Her bone broth way of life (I actually don't like to call it a diet) is a game-changer.

Now, Dr. Kellyann is back with *Dr. Kellyann's Cleanse and Reset*. I love that she recognizes that we all fall off track at times. She honestly admits that it happens to her, too, and she makes you feel hopeful instead of discouraged. Her plan is doable, sprinkled with her sense of humor, and easy to follow. If you are in need of restoration, inspiration, and invigoration, today is your lucky day, because you have just completed step one: you are holding this book in your hands, and you are about to embark on an incredible life-changing journey. It is an enormous honor to introduce you to Dr. Kellyann!

Elyse Walker

Owner, elysewalker and TOWNE by elysewalker

Fashion director of FWRD by elysewalker

PART 1

What My Cleanse and Reset Did for Me . . . and What It Can Do for You

Chapter 1

Why I Created This Cleanse—for ME

I want to tell you a story, but it's a little embarrassing—okay, *really* embarrassing—especially for a weight-loss and anti-aging specialist who's been helping patients get healthy for more than twenty years. However, I'm going to tell you anyway.

Why? Because, right now, I know you're not the "you" that you want to be. You desperately want to lose weight, to look better, and to *feel* better. And I want you to know that I've been there, too. Boy, have I.

You see, this cleanse is going to do amazing things for you, but I actually created it because *I'm* the one who needed it big-time. That's because I'm just human, and sometimes I blow it . . . I really screw up. And I blew it spectacularly a little while ago.

My Wake-Up Call

Normally, I take good care of myself. I really do practice what I preach—I exercise, get plenty of sleep, eat a natural diet, do all the right stuff. As a result, I'm slim and super-healthy . . . or at least I *was*.

In 2017, I let everything slide. I was running nonstop. I was writing a book. I was flying from coast to coast every week. I was seeing patients. Doing TV appearances. Running a business. Stressing out, losing sleep, and skipping workouts.

If you're in good shape, which I was at the start of 2017, you can get away with this kind of stuff for a while. But keep it up long enough, and your body will tell you, "What in the *world* do you think you're doing? Pay attention to ME!"

In my case, I ignored the early warning signs. I was putting on pounds, my skin looked like hell, my eyes were dull and sunken, and my energy level hovered near zero. I was wearing three pairs of Spanx to smooth out my butt and thighs when I went on TV. (It's true that the camera puts on ten pounds, and they're in all the wrong places.) Yet I still kept running.

Then my body finally sent me a message I *couldn't* ignore.

It was the fall of 2017. I was on an American Airlines flight from Los Angeles to New York. I'd felt tired and unwell all day, and suddenly I knew something was very, very wrong.

I became dizzy—so dizzy. It was as if I were in a tunnel being sucked away from reality. I was sweating profusely, and my heart was doing some weird kind of calisthenics.

All I knew was one thing: I was going down.

I turned to the passenger next to me and said, "I think I'm going to pass out. My name is Dr. Kellyann Petrucci, I don't take any medications, and I don't have any illnesses that I know of. Please get the flight attendant."

The next thing I knew, I was on the floor looking up at a flight attendant who was packing ice around my back and head and asking, "Are you okay? Are you okay?" As the flight crew dragged me back to the galley, I drifted in and out of consciousness, hearing the attendant call urgently for any medical professionals on board. Even though I was in a different world, I remember thinking, *What have I gotten myself into this time?*

(Okay, little digression here. Did you know that even in a situation like this, there are bright spots? Well, as I'm lying there, fading in and out, I hear one of the flight attendants saying, "That can't be her. It says on the passenger manifest that she's fifty-two. This woman is *not* fifty-two!" So, yeah. I'm lying on the floor of an airplane, feeling like I'm gonna die . . . but even half dead, at least I don't look my age. Woohoo.)

Anyway . . . back to the story. After the plane landed, they put me in a wheelchair and told me I needed to get checked out—basically saying, "No arguments." (They were already on to me.)

I wound up in a hospital, and then in a clinic. I was anemic. I was exhausted. I was both physically and emotionally drained. I'd gained twenty pounds, which is a HUGE weight gain when you're five-foot-nothing like me. My hormones were totally out of whack. I was a mess.

Sure, maybe I looked younger than my age (I love you, flight attendant!), but I still looked *terrible*. And to make matters worse, it was time to start promoting my brand-new book.

What's more, I didn't just look terrible; I *felt* terrible. And I suddenly realized that I'd felt that way for a long time, even though I was meeting wonderful people and having great experiences. I should have been having a blast, but instead I felt numb and disconnected. That's not "me," because by nature I'm a happy-go-lucky Italian girl with a big zest for life.

I realized that I needed a reset—and I needed it fast. I needed to reset my metabolism, my hormones, and even my mind. I needed to "push the compost button." Clean house. Take out the trash. Get my life back.

I needed RESTORATION.

As they say: "Physician, heal thyself."

Getting "Myself" Back

Right then, I went to work creating the cleanse detailed here. I knew that it needed to be incredibly powerful, because I was in deep trouble.

I knew that it needed to be *quick*, because I was sick and tired of feeling sick and tired (and fat). And I knew that it had to be simple, doable, and comfortable, because I was at the breaking point and couldn't handle any more stress.

I distilled into this plan every bit of knowledge I've gained over two decades. I loaded it with cell-cleansing, metabolism-boosting, fat-burning superfoods. Then I experimented until I got it just right.

What happened? Within days, I started feeling like "myself" again. My belly slimmed down, I lost the bloat, I got my energy back, the dark circles under my eyes went away, and I started feeling *happy* again. I'd jump-started my journey back to health, and now I was on a roll.

I was so excited about my plan that I started trying it out on my patients. Like me, they loved the results they got—both the weight loss and the energy and mood lift. They loved how they looked: younger, sexier, more vibrant. And they loved how they went from feeling depleted to feeling restored.

In short, I know that this cleanse can help you take back your life because it helped me take back mine—and now it's changing my patients' lives as well. What's more, it's fast, simple, and stress-free. (Because the last thing you need is more stress, right? I'm just not going to do that to you.)

So ask yourself: Are you exhausted, overweight, and feeling sad? Then this is *your* wake-up call. You can ignore it until you have a crisis, like I did, or you can take action right NOW.

Take it from someone who learned the hard way. Your body is telling you that it's time to hit the reset button—to pay attention—and it's easier than you think. You can *restore* yourself. Soon, I'll tell you exactly how to do it—but first, let's see just how much your body is craving a cleanse.

Take My Quick Cleanse Quiz

You can benefit from my cleanse even if you're at the top of your game right now. That's because it'll make your energy soar, smooth your skin, and sweep away toxins. In fact, I now do the cleanse four times a year, at the start of each season, to make sure I keep looking and feeling my best.

However, if you're less than perfectly healthy, you may *desperately* need this cleanse . . . just as I did when I crashed and burned. Here's a quick test to see how many cries for help your body is sending you.

Do You Need This Cleanse?

1. Are you gaining weight, especially around your belly?
2. Do you put on pounds easily and have trouble taking them off?
3. Have you gained ten pounds or more over the past few years?
4. Are you frequently bloated?
5. Do you often suffer from other gastrointestinal problems such as constipation or diarrhea?
6. Are you frequently tired?
7. Do you sleep badly?
8. Do you crave sleep?
9. Do you wake up feeling unrefreshed?
10. Do you experience a severe afternoon slump?
11. Do you feel like you are less strong and energetic than you used to be?
12. Do you feel that you're aging more quickly than you should?
13. Is your skin dry, or are you developing fine lines or wrinkles?
14. Is your skin blotchy or dull?
15. Do you have psoriasis or eczema?
16. Are your eyes red or dull?
17. Is your hair thin or lifeless?
18. Are your fingernails dry and brittle?
19. Are you frequently exposed to toxins from smog, traffic, household cleansers, or other sources?

20. Do you frequently eat non-organic fruits and vegetables or non-pastured meat and eggs?
21. Do you drink unfiltered water?
22. Do you frequently get sick?
23. When you get sick, do you have trouble "bouncing back"?
24. Do you have autoimmune problems?
25. Are you frequently angry or unhappy?
26. Are you often anxious?
27. Do you frequently experience "brain fog"?
28. Do you enjoy sex less than you used to?
29. Do you enjoy your friends and family less than you used to?
30. Do you enjoy life less than you used to?

Now, count up your number of "yes" answers. Here's how to score your results:

If your score is 10 or above, your body is screaming that it needs help.

If your score is 5 to 9, you're entering the danger zone and it's time to stop problems before they get worse.

If your score is 0 to 4, you're in far better shape than most people—congratulations! You need the cleanse only if you want to take your well-being to an even higher level.

Take a hard look at your score. If it reveals that you're crashing and burning—or that you're just getting by when you want to be awesome—it's decision time right now.

If you're sick of being fat, tired, and sad, then decide that now is the time to take your life back.

You matter—so here's to becoming the best, happiest you that you can be. Here's to feeling better than you have in years, or maybe in your entire life.

Decide, commit, and go. Let's do this!

This cleanse is an ideal choice for anyone who wants to slim down and get healthier quickly. However, if you fall into one of the categories below, you should postpone the diet for now or only do the diet under medical supervision.

Are you pregnant or nursing? If that's the case, wait until later to do your cleanse. When you're eating for two, you'll need more food than you get on this diet. However, this cleanse is a fantastic way to take off those extra baby pounds later on! It'll also help you restore nutrients lost while you're nurturing your little one.

Are you diabetic, or are you taking drugs to lower your blood sugar? This cleanse will lower your blood glucose, and that's a very good thing. However, if you're taking insulin or a drug like metformin, you need to be careful not to become hypoglycemic. Get your doctor's approval before doing the cleanse and check your blood sugar numbers frequently each day.

Do you have other chronic health problems? Get your doctor's okay to do the cleanse and ask if you'll need to adjust any of your medications.

Are you taking a blood thinner? This cleanse contains lots of healthy greens. These greens are rich in vitamin K, which can interfere with anticlotting drugs, so check with your doctor to make sure it's safe for you. If not, you can swap out your evening soup for plain bone broth and replace your green smoothies with shakes containing fewer veggies.

Are you under eighteen? If so, make sure your parents and your doctor say it's fine for you to do the cleanse.

Do you have a history of an eating disorder? Check with

your doctor and make sure this cleanse will be safe for you to do.

Do you have an illness right now or are you recovering from an injury? If so, your body needs to direct all of its resources toward getting you well. Hold off on the cleanse until you're better ... I'll wait for you!

Chapter 2

The Science Behind My Cleanse and Reset

I know you can't wait to heal your body on this cleanse, and I'm eager for you to get started, too. But if you're tempted to skip this chapter and head right for the cleanse, bear with me for just a few more pages.

Before you begin your cleanse, I want to give you the lowdown on it. I believe that knowledge is power, so I want you to know exactly what my cleanse will do for you and why I included every single element.

There's a lot of science in this chapter, not because I want your eyes to glaze over, but because it will help you understand why this new way of cleansing is so important—and so different from the cleanses you've done in the past.

What This Cleanse Is—and Isn't

First of all, I want to tell you what I mean by a *cleanse*. Most people think that cleanses are all about depletion and deprivation. But this cleanse is going to *build you up*, not break you down.

After years of being in the health field, witnessing thousands of patients' experiences, and having my own personal experiences, I've seen the good, the bad, and the ugly when it comes to cleanses. I've learned the hard way, and I know what a cleanse should and shouldn't do.

When you finish my cleanse, you're going to be renewed, not drained. You're going to feel light on your feet, not weak and tired. You're going to have the energy of a teenager—you know, "tiger blood."

That's because this cleanse is going to fire up your cellular matrix—the fluid around your cells—by *saturating* your body with energizing nutrients. You see, that's the name of the game: loading yourself up with all the right stuff.

At the same time, these nutrients are going to gently cleanse your cells of toxins. My patients frequently tell me, "You know, Dr. Kellyann, somehow my insides feel *clean*." You'll feel like you just went through one of those luxury car washes, got scrubbed and buffed, and came out shiny and new.

On this cleanse, you're going to pamper your body, not punish it. I like to say, "It's not just about how you heal—it's about how you feel," and this cleanse will make you feel like a brand-new you.

And that's not all; you're also going to *look* like a brand-new you. On some cleanses, you wind up looking drawn and unhealthy. This cleanse is going to tighten your skin, so instead of feeling "stringy" and loose, you'll end up looking young and sculpted.

Why You Need This Cleanse

If you're in the same place I was when I hit the wall—tired, sick, sad, and gaining weight—it's because your body is beginning to fail. And it's beginning to fail because it's not getting what it needs.

In fact, even if you're trying to eat right, you could be cheating your body of nutrients it needs. In one study, John Berardi, PhD, analyzed the diets of more than five hundred students as part of his master's degree project. Even though the students were taking a class in exercise and nutrition, Berardi found that "only about 10 to 15% of them met all of their dietary needs." Note that these were *health-conscious people consciously trying to eat right*.[1]

Another study[2] analyzed the diets of twenty people—fourteen were health-conscious athletes—all of them eating what they thought were good diets. The scientist conducting the study reported, "All of these dietary analyses fell short of the recommended 100% RDA micronutrient level from food alone." That's right: *all* of them.

What's more, these studies looked only at the nutrients for which we have recommended daily amounts—not many more, such as the thousands of phytonutrients that our cells crave. These powerful plant chemicals include:

- Anthocyanins, which give foods like berries, red onions, and pomegranates their beautiful color—and which protect your skin from sun damage,[3] help to prevent cancer,[4] and reduce your risk of becoming obese or diabetic.[5]
- Lutein and zeaxanthin, which keep the maculae of your eyes healthy, helping to prevent blindness due to macular degeneration.[6]
- Lycopene, a potent antioxidant and inflammation fighter that can lower your risk for cancer,[7] reduce your blood pressure,[8] and even lower your stroke risk by up to 59%.[9]
- Resveratrol, which helps to give berries, grapes, and red wine their beautiful color—and which can slow the effects of aging by protecting your mitochondria (the "power plants" of your cells).[10]
- Quercetin, which helps to strengthen a "leaky gut" (more on this later), reducing chronic inflammation.[11]

The bottom line? Each day, your deficit of phytonutrients—as well as vitamins, minerals, and other nutrients—increases a tiny bit. So over time, your body starts to starve for nutrients even when you're doing all the right things.

If you're stressed out, losing sleep, grabbing fast food, and neglecting yourself, like I was before I collapsed, you're in even bigger trouble. That's because you need big doses of nutrients to heal yourself—but you're not getting them because your gut is sick and inflamed and your metabolism is sluggish. That cellular matrix I talked about earlier is no longer working for you—it's working against you, because it's a toxic swamp. So you get sicker and sicker and sicker.

This is what landed me on the floor of an airplane cabin. And it's what's going to make you crash and burn if you're in bad shape and you don't take action by *loading* your cells with nutrients. You don't need just a trickle of these lifesaving nutrients right now—you need a flood.

What's more, you need to load up on *every* crucial healing nutrient your body is craving. Shorting your cells of even a few essential nutrients can wipe you out. For example:

- Too little potassium will make you feel weak, anxious, and bloated.
- Too little magnesium will make you tired, "brain fogged," and achy, and cause headaches and muscle cramps.
- Too little vitamin A will make your thyroid hormones wonky, causing you to pack on pounds.
- Too little vitamin C will shut down your collagen production line, aging your skin and hurting your gut.
- Too little zinc can make your hair thin and make you more prone to infections.
- Too little folic acid can make you feel exhausted, cause a racing heart and shortness of breath, and lead to headaches.
- Too little healthy fat will stop your body from absorbing fat-soluble vitamins.
- Too little blood-building iron will make you weak and make your hair thin and fragile.

So it's not enough to supplement your diet with a few nutrients. You need to get every major player in the healing game. Even missing a small number of nutrients can be a concern.

Loading your body with nutrients is especially critical if you're battling a weight problem. Research shows obese adults have a lower intake of micronutrients than people who aren't overweight,[12] and these nutritional deficiencies can increase the risk of developing diabetes.[13] (For more on this topic, read "Are You at Risk for Developing Diabetes?" on the Resources page of my website at drkellyann.com/cleansebook.)

On this cleanse, we're going to bathe your cells in hundreds of vitamins, minerals, and phytonutrients. And we're going to load you with *combinations* of nutrients—for instance, the healthy fats you'll get along with big doses of vitamins, minerals, and phytonutrients—that work synergistically to build you up cell by cell.

Note: To make sure you get the key nutrients you need while still giving your gut a rest from solid food, consider taking a daily multivitamin and multimineral supplement during your cleanse. If multivitamin and multimineral supplements don't sit well with you, then be sure to get some sunshine every day (for vitamin D), include some sea veggies in your soups or green smoothies (for iodine, zinc, selenium, and molybdenum), and consider taking a B-complex supplement. Mushrooms are a good source of selenium and (if they've been exposed to sunlight) vitamin D, so work them into your soups as well.

In addition, unlike many cleanses, my cleanse is going to load your body with a key macronutrient—clean *protein*—in the forms of collagen and bone broth. You may think that a cleanse is supposed to be just green juice or water because there's a myth that you need to cut protein out of a cleanse for it to work. In reality, *this is the biggest reason why other cleanses can leave you looking haggard and feeling terrible.* Your body needs the amino acids in protein to heal your cells, repair your joints, banish your bloat, optimize your immune function, make your skin and hair beautiful, and create a strong gut wall.

In addition, your body needs amino acids to "take out the trash" that's clogging your cells. In particular, it needs the amino acid *glycine*, which plays a key role in one of your body's detoxification pathways.

And here's another thing to understand. One reason that many cleanses cut out protein is to allow your gut to rest. However, collagen and bone broth are clean, allergen-free proteins that are easy for your body to digest because they're in liquid form. These gentle foods feed your body the amino acids you need while still giving your gut "down time" for recovery. In addition, they help to prevent those cravings and crashes you may have experienced in the past.

Finally, a cleanse that allows you to rotate shakes, green smoothies, and soups works far better than an all-green-drinks cleanse because typical juice and smoothie cleanses overload your body with sugar—and sugar makes your cells wonky. One cleanse that I researched recommended drinking six juice drinks per day, and each drink contained 35 to 50 grams of sugar from fruits. That's not much healthier than a soda cleanse would be! On this cleanse, you'll get a very limited amount of sugar while you supply your body with lots of clean protein.

You don't want to overload your body with sugar on a cleanse because sugar does the very opposite of healing your body. When you eat sugar, it reacts with the proteins or fats in your body to form destructive compounds called *advanced glycation end products*, or AGEs. These nasty molecules stiffen your tissues and inflame your body. Excess AGEs are linked to everything from diabetes to Alzheimer's disease, and they also prematurely age your skin, leading to wrinkles and age spots.

In addition, sugar increases your risk for cancer. A 2016 study on mice by researchers at MD Anderson Cancer Center found that high-sugar diets can significantly raise your risk for both cancer development and metastasis.[14]

And here's another alarming new finding: a diet that's high in sugar shortens your telomeres. These are the tips on the ends of your chromosomes—sort of like the aglets on the ends of shoelaces—and the shorter they are, the faster you age and the more vulnerable you are to diseases like cancer. In a 2018 study, scientists reported that children who drink lots of sugary beverages already have shorter telomeres than their non-sugar-swigging peers by *the age of three!*[15] In a 2014 study of adults, researchers at the University of California at San Francisco determined that based on the rate at which telomeres typically shorten with chronological age, daily consumption of a 20-ounce soda is equivalent to an average of 4.6 years of telomere shortening—comparable to the effects of smoking.[16]

Clearly, a sugar-loaded cleanse can worsen your health, not make it better. And in the end, it can pack pounds on you rather than take them off.

So if you've tried juice cleanses in the past and they let you down, I want you to understand that this cleanse is different. This time, instead of loading your body with sugar, you're going to be combining the phytonutrients from greens with healthy fats and clean protein from collagen and bone broth—and this triple punch of nutrients is going to lift you up, not tear you down.

My Three Cleanse Goals

When I created my cleanse, I set down three non-negotiable goals for it. Now, it's time for you to achieve these same goals. Here's what you're going to do on this cleanse:

Rest. You're going to allow your body to take a break from the hard work of processing food. This "holiday" will allow your leaky gut—and it's pretty much guaranteed that you have one, if you're not feeling up to par (more on this in a bit)—to seal and heal itself.

Restore. Right now, your body is depleted of many nutrients it needs to repair itself. When you push all those nutrients into your cellular matrix, you're going to give it all of the resources it needs to undo the damage that's making you feel old and sick.

Revitalize. If you're fatigued all the time right now, this cleanse is going to re-energize you. That's because it's rich in foods that power up your cells, and it cuts out foods that make them sluggish.

These are big promises, I know. But I'm 100% confident in making them because I know this plan works. I initially created it to save my own life, so I wasn't kidding around.

I know that this cleanse can do for you what it did for me. In just days, it can take you from being half-dead to back in action. It transformed my life, and it's doing the same for my patients. Now, it's time to put it to work for you.

How My Cleanse Works

I can sum up this cleanse in just six words: *push nutrients in and toxins out*. Here are the five ways we're going to do this.

1. Hydrolyzed Collagen

Collagen is the structural protein that holds your body together. (Think of it as Mother Nature's glue.) More than 30% of your body is collagen—but if you're over twenty, you're losing 1% of that collagen every year. This is one of the biggest reasons why you're feeling old, tired, and wiped out.

When you lose collagen, your skin gets weak and starts to wrinkle and sag. Your butt and thighs develop "cottage cheese" bumps. Your hair gets brittle, and your fingernails break easily. While you're aging on the outside, you're aging on the inside at the same time, because your internal collagen stores are running dry. Your gut gets inflamed, your bones weaken, and your joints hurt. You gain weight, and you lose muscle.

Luckily, there's a simple solution: get that collagen back in your life. You'll do this every day on the cleanse by adding collagen powder to your shakes and green smoothies and drinking soups made from bone broth (which is rich in the building blocks of collagen).

Let's start by talking about the collagen powder. The collagen you'll put in your shakes and green smoothies is *hydrolyzed collagen*, also known as *collagen peptides* or *collagen hydrolysate*. During the process of hydrolyzation, large molecules of collagen break down into smaller units called *peptides*. These peptides contain high concentrations of the amino acids that build collagen in a form your body can easily assimilate and use.

Here's what this superfood does for you:

Superpower #1: It accelerates your fat loss and protects lean muscle. This is a truly beautiful thing. If you've dieted a lot, you know that much of the weight you lose is muscle mass, not belly fat. So instead of looking strong and sculpted after your diet, you're wrecked.

What you need is a magic bullet that ramps up your fat loss while it protects your lean muscle mass—and on my cleanse, you'll get one. It's an amino acid called *glycine*, which your body will get from collagen.

A recent study demonstrated the fat-melting, lean-mass-preserving effects of glycine. In it, researchers fattened mice and then put them on a weight-loss diet. One group of mice got supplemental glycine, while a control group got a different amino acid.

By the end of the study, the glycine-treated mice lost 14% more whole-body fat mass and 27% less lean mass than the control mice.[17] These are amazing numbers, and they show why juice-only cleanses can't achieve the same results as this cleanse. Remember: juice cleanses make you feel stringy and loose, while a cleanse that's rich in collagen makes you feel rebuilt.

Superpower #2: It makes your cells more sensitive to insulin. To lose pounds and heal your body, you need to convince your cells to love the hormone insulin. Once again, you're going to reach for glycine-rich collagen. Here's why.

Insulin carries sugar to your cells. When your cells are insulin-sensitive, they accept this sugar and burn it for energy.

However, if your blood sugar is constantly spiking—which happens if you eat lots of carbs, even if they're supposedly "healthy" carbs like whole grains—your cells get stuffed with sugar. When this happens, they start to turn insulin and its cargo of sugar away. (This is called *insulin resistance*.) This sugar goes back to your liver, which turns it into fat. So you pack on belly fat because you're storing that energy instead of burning it.

How can you lower your insulin resistance? First, cut down on carbs (which you'll do on this cleanse)—and then feed your body glycine.

In a recent experiment, researchers fed rats sugar to make them insulin-resistant. Giving them glycine after this sugar load ramped up their insulin sensitivity (as well as lowering their levels of oxidative stress, or damage to cells caused by destructive molecules).[18]

In a related study, scientists gave healthy people a dose of glycine along with a dose of glucose. The glycine reduced the participants' increase in blood glucose to *half* of the rise seen when glucose alone was consumed. Insulin levels rose only a little in the glycine group, leading the scientists to speculate that glycine stimulates the release of another hormone that helps insulin to work better.[19]

Superpower #3: It pulls toxins from your body. Because this is a cleanse and not a harsh detox, you're going to *gently* flush toxins out of your system with nutrients—and collagen will be a big part of your cleanup crew. The proline and glycine in collagen are both potent detoxifiers on their own. In addition, glycine is a building block of glutathione, a molecular powerhouse that grabs on to toxins and whisks them out of your body in urine or bile.

Remember what you're going to do on this cleanse: push nutrients in and toxins out. And glycine is a big player in this game.

Glycine: NOT Nonessential!

Doctors call glycine a "nonessential" amino acid because we once believed that your body could make plenty of it on its own. However, we now know better. In reality, unless you're very young, you're in ideal health, and you eat an ideal diet, there's a good chance that you're glycine-deficient.[20] That's a big reason for loading up on glycine, and it's why even after your cleanse, I want you to keep drinking glycine-rich collagen drinks and bone broth every day. You will become obsessed (in a good way) when you see the changes to your body and skin!

Superpower #4: It lowers your inflammation and strengthens your gut. The glycine in collagen is an inflammation-fighting master, and one of its most important jobs is to prevent or heal damage to your gut wall.[21] The healthier and less inflamed your gut is, the faster you're going to heal your body. (I'll talk about this much more in the next section.)

Superpower #5: It beautifies your skin. This cleanse is about making you stronger, healthier, and more vibrant—and as a big plus, it's going to make you more beautiful as well. That's because collagen firms and smooths your skin like a tight pair of jeans, blasting your wrinkles. When you mainline it to your cells, the results will amaze you.

In one double-blind, placebo-controlled study,[22] for example, women between the ages of forty-five and sixty-five received either a collagen peptide supplement or a placebo for eight weeks. The results were nothing short of astonishing.

At the end of the treatment period, the group taking collagen experienced an average 20.1% reduction in eye wrinkles when compared to the placebo group—and the maximum reduction observed was

49.9%! Four weeks after the treatment stopped, the collagen group still showed an average 11.5% reduction in wrinkles.

In addition, at the end of the study, the researchers detected a 65% increase in procollagen (a building block of collagen) and an 18% increase in elastin, a protein that makes your skin "bounce back" when it's stretched. These are stunning results—better than anything the most expensive wrinkle creams on the market can achieve.

2. Bone Broth-Based Soups

Now, let's talk about the other source of amino acids on your cleanse—bone broth, the magic food I call "liquid gold." Every day, you'll be drinking soup made from this fabulous food.

Lots of my patients call me the Bone Broth Doctor. And I admit it: I'm obsessed with bone broth. In fact, I was one of the pioneers of the modern bone broth movement.

People said two things to me when this movement first started. The first was "yuck"—because they had no idea how good bone broth is—and the second was "Bone broth is going to be a short-lived fad." But I knew it was going to last because bone broth is one of *the most amazing healing foods on the planet*.

In every traditional culture, all around the world, people turn to bone broth when they need to heal and restore themselves. When a piece of folk wisdom is this universal, you can assume there's hard science behind it. And indeed, research shows that bone broth is serious medicine—every bit as powerful as traditional healers believe.

If you're not familiar with bone broth, it's not at all like broth from a can, or even regular broth made from scratch. Instead, it's made from bones that you simmer for hours and hours, pulling the deep nutrition out of the bones. Because it's rich in glycine, it gives you many of the same benefits as collagen—and here are even more reasons why this broth is such powerful medicine.

THE GELATIN IN BONE BROTH HEALS YOUR GUT.
Bone broth is rich in gelatin, which is basically cooked collagen. This gelatin reduces inflammation in your gut, which is a huge key to healing yourself. Here's why:

These days, we know that *chronic inflammation* is the biggest cause of obesity and age-related illnesses. In addition, we know that this body-wide inflammation starts in the gut. This is one of the most important principles to understand if you want to stay healthy and fight aging.

The first thing to know about chronic inflammation is that it's very different from *acute* inflammation. When you cut a finger or catch the flu, your immune system rushes into action to fight off germs. That's a very good thing, and it's temporary.

Chronic inflammation, in contrast, is like a forest fire that never goes out. It poisons your cells, and it makes you sick and fat.

This internal forest fire starts in your gut's *microbiome*, an ecosystem containing trillions of microbes. (I like to say that you're a big bag of bugs.) These microbes do everything from digesting your food to putting the brakes on your immune system. When they're healthy, you're healthy—and when they're not, things get ugly really fast. Here's what happens:

- Environmental insults—that is, environment-related factors, such as stress, antibiotic use, toxins, or a poor diet—throw your gut bacteria out of whack, letting bad bugs gain a foothold or letting normally beneficial bugs overmultiply.
- This local inflammation damages the wall of your intestine, causing little holes to open up in it. (We call this a *leaky gut*.)
- Toxins and undigested food molecules escape through these holes into your bloodstream, where your immune system labels them as enemies and goes on the attack. This assault damages your own cells in a case of "friendly fire."

This nonstop attack leads to body-wide inflammation that makes you gain weight like crazy. In addition, research links it to type 2 diabetes.[23]

When you drink bone broth, it puts out this internal fire. The gelatin in the broth soothes and heals your gut, like rubbing aloe vera on a sunburn. Your intestinal wall heals, becoming rock-solid. Toxins and undigested food stop escaping—so your immune system stands down, your inflammation vanishes, and extra pounds melt away.

For more on building a glowing gut, see my article on "Keeping Your Gut Healthy" on the Resources page of my website at drkellyann.com/cleansebook.

How Inflamed Are You?

You may be experiencing many signs and symptoms of chronic inflammation without even realizing it. To get an idea of how inflamed your body is, take this quick quiz.

Do you have a large amount of belly fat?
Are your blood sugar levels higher than they should be?
Do you have gum disease?
Do you have joint aches and pains?
Do you suffer from "brain fog," anxiety, or depression?
Do you have frequent headaches?
Do you have chronic digestive problems such as bloating, constipation, or diarrhea?
Are you frequently fatigued?
Do you have eczema or psoriasis?
Do you suffer from an autoimmune disease?

The more "yes" answers you have, the more likely it is that chronic inflammation is taking a huge toll on your body and mind.

THE NUTRIENTS IN BONE BROTH HEAL YOUR JOINTS.

Bone broth is rich in glucosamine and chondroitin, which doctors often prescribe to ease joint pain. One study found that these two nutrients eased the pain caused by osteoarthritis as effectively as the prescription drug Celebrex.[24] In addition, bone broth is brimming with hyaluronic acid, which helps to lubricate your joints. So it doesn't surprise me when patients call me up just to say, "I can't believe it, Kellyann—my knees don't hurt anymore!"

THE GELATIN IN BONE BROTH STRENGTHENS YOUR HAIR AND NAILS.

Your grandmother was right when she told you to eat gelatin—and the scientific research backs her up. One two-part study found that eating 14 grams of gelatin daily increased hair diameter by an average of 9.3% in the first part of the study and 11.3% in the second part. Seventy percent of participants had thicker hair by the end of the study, and the greatest increase seen was an amazing 45%![25] Similarly, researchers have known for decades that gelatin can make your nails stronger and improve defects.[26]

Finally, bone broth isn't just good medicine . . . it's delicious. It's rich and satisfying, and it feeds your body deep nutrition that keeps your hunger at bay for hours. It truly is a meal in a mug, and my patients are *amazed* at how it stops cravings in their tracks. They keep drinking it long after their cleanses because they discover that there's no better way to curtail hunger for long periods than by sipping bone broth.

Bone broth and collagen are two of the healthiest foods you can eat. A few people, however, have a reaction to bone broth or supplements containing collagen. These people experience symptoms such as headaches, digestive upsets, heart palpitations, and skin flushing. When this happens, a likely culprit is *histamine intolerance*, a problem that affects about 1% of people.

Histamine is a neurotransmitter that plays an important role in keeping your immune system, your digestion, and your nervous system working right. Many foods are high in histamine, promote the release of histamine, or limit its breakdown. These foods include shellfish, nuts, chocolate, citrus fruits, tomatoes, black and green teas, spinach, fermented foods, collagen, and bone broth.

For the vast majority of people, the amount of histamine in a food simply isn't an issue. If your system is working right, it immediately inactivates any histamine you don't need, using two enzymes called DAO and HNMT, and that's the end of the story.

Sometimes, however, things go wrong. A number of factors, from genetic mutations to medical conditions like Crohn's disease, can lead to high levels of histamine. In some cases, the only solution may be to stay on a histamine intolerance diet forever.

However—and I want to emphasize this—*the most common problem in people with histamine intolerance is a sick, leaky gut.* In these cases, healing the gut may make histamine issues vanish.

There are two reasons for this. First, if you have an inflamed gut, DAO—which does much of its work in the intestine—can't do its job right. As a result, it won't break down enough histamine. Second, if your gut is leaky, histamines can escape through your gut wall, triggering a violent immune system reaction.

The solution is obvious: fix your leaky gut, and DAO can rein in those histamines. In addition, histamines will stop escaping into your blood stream and setting off your immune system's alarms.

So that's the *why* behind this healing strategy. Now, let's get to the *how*. Here's the way to go about building a rock-solid gut if you have histamine issues:

- Cut grains, sugar, soy, dairy, and artificial ingredients from your diet. All of these damage your gut.
- Initially, avoid even healthy foods that are high in histamines. (It's easy to find lists of them online.) Remember, however, that the histamine content of a food may vary depending on its age and other factors. Also, experts don't always agree on which foods belong on the high-histamine list, so you may need to do a little experimenting.
- Eat egg yolks and fresh, lean meat and poultry. If you have leftovers, freeze them immediately. (The histamine level of meat increases over time.)
- Eat fresh fruits, fresh vegetables, and healthy fats that aren't on the high-histamine list.
- Rather than drinking bone broth, drink meat broth (which cooks for only a few hours). It contains fewer histamines, and it'll still help to heal your gut. When you make your broth, use or freeze it quickly. You can also substitute vegetable broth (see my vegetarian option on page 185).
- Supplement wisely. Take vitamin C, which helps degrade histamine; vitamin B_6, which helps DAO do its job; zinc, which is a powerful anti-inflammatory nutrient; and quercetin, which is a natural antihistamine.
- Avoid alcohol.
- Exercise, get enough sleep, and ease your stress with meditation, yoga, Tai Chi, or breathing exercises.

After you've given your gut several months to heal, try introducing small amounts of high-histamine foods. With luck, you'll discover that you can handle them just fine. And as a result—hurray—you can start enjoying all the benefits of skin-healing, fat-melting collagen and bone broth!

In the meantime, if you want to do your cleanse without including bone broth, collagen, or even meat broth in your diet, check out my vegetarian and vegan modifications on page 67. These will work just fine for you.

---

3. Fresh Veggies and Fruits

Each day on this cleanse, you're going to fill your body with a rainbow of veggies and fruits in your soups, shakes, and green smoothies. These will load you up with hundreds of phytochemicals that brighten your eyes, build strong skin, energize your cells, and "take out the trash" by flushing out toxins.

The veggies and fruits you eat on your cleanse will fill you with fiber to regulate your GI tract, banishing bloat and clearing up constipation. They'll also lower your blood sugar because fiber increases the thickness of your intestinal contents, slowing down carbohydrate digestion and glucose absorption.

In addition, this fiber is going to make your gut bugs very happy. That's because they can ferment soluble fiber to create a short-chain fatty acid called *butyrate*, which plays a key role in healing a leaky gut.

As researcher Alanna Collen explains in her book *10% Human*, "It is our microbes that decide how much to turn up the volume on the genes that make the protein chains of the gut wall. Butyrate is their messenger. The more butyrate they can produce, the more protein chains our genes churn out, and the tighter the gut wall."[27]

And creating a rock-solid gut is just one of butyrate's effects. It's also anti-inflammatory, and it helps to protect against colon cancer[28]—

a disease that strikes 140,000 people in the United States each year. In addition, butyrate increases insulin sensitivity and promotes fat-burning.[29]

What's more, the fruits and veggies you'll eat on your cleanse have benefits that go beyond fiber. They'll also help you lose weight because the nutrients in them satisfy your hunger and slash your cravings. In addition, they'll ramp up your levels of nitric oxide, a molecule that relaxes your arteries, lowers your blood pressure, builds muscle, and even makes sex better by enhancing both pleasure and performance. (See, I've got your back.)

In fact, every single fruit and veggie you eat on this cleanse will bring something to the party. I know you already know that fruits and vegetables are good for you—yada, yada—but did you know that they also have individual superpowers that can help make you so nutrient-dense that you're bionic? It's true! Here are some examples:

Beets. These beautiful red root vegetables contain *betalains*, which have antioxidant and anti-inflammatory properties. Research shows that one type of betalain, called *betanin*, inhibits the development of lung cancer[30] and may help fight skin and liver cancer as well.[31]

Celery. You've probably heard a lot about celery juice already because it's gotten its share of good press. This veggie is rich in *luteolin*, a phytochemical with cancer-fighting properties.[32] It's also a good source of an anti-inflammatory compound called *butylphthalide* and a potent cancer fighter called *apigenin*.[33]

Citrus fruits. These delicious fruits contain a phytochemical called *hesperidin*, which helps your blood vessels stay healthy and aids in preventing varicose veins.

Cruciferous veggies. These veggies are rich in sulfur-containing compounds called *glucosinolates*, which break down when you chew and digest them into biologically active compounds that can inhibit bladder, breast, colon, liver, lung, and stomach cancer.[34] Cruciferous veggies include arugula, bok choy, broccoli, Brussels sprouts, cabbage, cauliflower, collard greens, horseradish, kale, radishes, turnip greens, watercress, and wasabi.

Grapefruit. This fruit is loaded with a chemical called *nootkatone*, which stimulates your metabolism and ramps up your fat burning. (Just make sure that if you're taking any medications, it's okay to add grapefruit or grapefruit juice to your diet.)

Pineapples. These fruits feed your body *bromelain*, which helps to lower inflammation, protect against blood clots, and fight cancer.

Raspberries. While many fruits and veggies contain the cholesterol-lowering, cancer-preventing phytochemical *ellagic acid*, raspberries have the highest amount of all.

Seaweed. Ocean veggies are rich in iodine, which is crucial when it comes to thyroid function. They're also denser in nutrients overall than land veggies are.

These individual superpowers help to explain why eating a cornucopia of fruits and veggies matters to your health. Check out these findings:

- One study of nearly 4,000 men and women found that two factors—eating lots of veggies *and* eating a greater variety of fruits and veggies—are independently beneficial in reducing the risk of type 2 diabetes. Even when the researchers controlled for the amount of produce people ate, each additional two-item-per-week increase in *variety* was associated with an 8% reduction in the incidence of type 2 diabetes.[35]
- A study by a different group of researchers came to the same conclusion when it comes to lung cancer: eating a greater variety of fruits and veggies lowers your risk, independently of how *many* you eat.[36]

So be adventurous with the fruits and veggies you use in your soups, shakes, and green smoothies. The more you switch things up, the more of these superpowers you'll put to work for you.

A Note About Fiber

Put simply, fiber is a carbohydrate that you can't digest—so it doesn't hike your blood sugar. There are two types of fiber, and both of them help to ramp up the benefits of your cleanse. Here they are:

Soluble fiber, which dissolves in water, helps to keep your blood sugar low and optimize your cholesterol. Foods rich in soluble fiber include apples, blueberries, citrus fruits, Brussels sprouts, leafy greens, and sweet potatoes.

Insoluble fiber, which doesn't dissolve in water, fights bloat and constipation. Foods rich in insoluble fibers include carrots, cucumbers, and tomatoes.

---

4. Healthy Fats

During your cleanse, you're going to get a good dose of healthy fats each day. Your body craves these fats, using them to make hormones, build bouncy cell walls that smooth out wrinkles, and give you energy. You also need them to make you happy and clear up brain fog—in fact, 60% of your brain is made of fat!

I know that nutritionists have scared you for years with the "fat makes you fat" myth, but we now know that it's just that: a myth. The truth is that good fats burn fat and make your body healthier at the same time. If you're fat-phobic and need convincing, here's what the research says:

- The A to Z Weight Loss Study lasted twelve months and involved more than three hundred overweight women. It compared four diets: Atkins (the lowest in carbs and highest in fat), Zone,

Ornish, and the LEARN diet. The women eating the Atkins diet lost *twice as much weight* as the women eating the other diets—and their cholesterol and blood pressure improved as well.[37]

- Another study compared the effects of the Paleo diet (which is rich in fats and low in carbs) to a standard low-fat diabetic diet on patients with type 2 diabetes. Researchers found that compared to the standard diabetes diet, the Paleo diet resulted in lower HbA1c levels (a long-term measure of blood sugar levels), lower triglyceride levels, lower blood pressure levels, and higher levels of HDL ("good") cholesterol. In addition, the high-fat, low-carb dieters lost more weight than the diabetic-diet group.[38]

- Cochrane, a highly respected health research group, reviewed low-glycemic and high-glycemic diets. (Low-glycemic diets are rich in fats and low in carbs, while high-glycemic diets are low in fats and high in carbs.) The group concluded, "Overweight or obese people on low-glycemic-index diets lost more weight and had more improvement in lipid profiles than those receiving comparison diets." What's more, the researchers found that people on the low-glycemic diets did as well as or better than those on calorie-controlled high-glycemic diets *even when the people on the low-glycemic diets got to eat as much as they wanted.*[39]

In short, good fats like olive oil, avocados, and coconut oil are **fat-burners,** not fat promoters. Eat the right fats in the right amounts, and you'll **lose** weight, not gain it. Moreover, as the studies show, these fats are good for your cholesterol, your blood pressure, and your blood sugar. And they fill you up, so you can go for long stretches without any cravings at all.

So during your cleanse (and afterward), eat healthy fats fearlessly. Your body will thank you.

5. Mini-Meals Comprised of Low-Carb Foods—and an Optional "Keto Push"

On this cleanse, while you won't actually be fasting, you'll be limiting your meals to small, easy-to-digest soups, shakes, and green smoothies. In addition, you're going to cut your carb intake way down.

As a result, you'll reduce your insulin levels dramatically—and that will make extra pounds around your belly fall off quickly. That fat is a witch's cauldron of toxic chemicals and fattening hormones, and melting it off will make your entire body not just slimmer but also healthier and happier.

And if you really, *really* want to rev up your fat burning, and you're not faint of heart, I have an optional bonus for you: a powerful one-day pre-cleanse jump-start I call the Keto Push. If you choose this option, you'll spend the day *before* your cleanse drinking nothing but water or bone broth (more on this later). After that, you'll jump right into the cleanse itself.

If you opt for the Keto Push, you'll start burning fat right out of the gate. That's because when you slash your carbs to a bare minimum, it helps to drive your body toward a state called *ketosis*, in which it burns a type of fat called *ketone bodies* rather than sugar for energy. This turns you into a fat-burning machine.

But remember: the Keto Push is *totally* optional, and you'll get amazing results (including weight loss) with or without it. It's an entirely personal decision, so do what works for you—either the five-day cleanse alone or the five-day cleanse preceded by the one-day Keto Push.

If you're currently following a keto plan, you can easily modify this entire cleanse to be keto-friendly. Simply do the Keto Push on the first day, and then on the following days eliminate the fruit and starchy veggies from your green smoothies, shakes, and soups. You'll find a list of keto-friendly recipes on page 52.

So, Are You In?

Now you know what my cleanse is going to do for you. It's going to *restore* you, not deplete you. It's going to *energize* you—not wipe you out. You're going to go into it sick and fat and old, and come out of it shiny and new.

So—are you game? Then I'll tell you exactly how this plan works—starting with your cleanse prep in Chapter 3.

PART 2

*How to Do
the Cleanse*

Chapter 3

Preparing for Your Cleanse

When you're taking a big step to improve your life, it's smart to prepare in advance—and that's why I want you to put all the pieces for success in place before you start your cleanse.

In this chapter, I'll tell you how to ready yourself, your friends and family, and your kitchen for your cleanse. Here's what I want you to do before Day 1.

1. Pick a date. Choose a time when your schedule is as light as possible. The fewer obligations you have, the easier it'll be to stick to your cleanse. In particular, try to avoid days when you have social events that involve food. (I mean, what could go wrong if you haven't had any sweets in three days and you come face-to-face with a five-tier mocha chocolate wedding cake? You get the idea.)

2. Think hard about why you're doing this. I always start any important project with the end in mind, and that's why I don't want you to jump into this cleanse on a whim. Instead, I want you to understand *why* you're undertaking it. Identifying your goals will help you stay strong and stop you from looking for an escape hatch.

So ask yourself: Are you sick and tired of being sick and tired? Are you burned out, depleted, sad, or feeling years older than you are? Or are you merely feeling "okay" rather than being the best you can be? No matter where you are on the scale, I think you'll realize that you need to take action.

Before you begin your cleanse, I want you to write down all of the reasons you're doing it. Post your list on your fridge or your bathroom mirror, where you'll see it every day during your cleanse. This will inspire you to stay the course even if things get challenging.

As human beings, we tend to do things in two steps. First, we imprint a desire in our mind. Second, we make that desire materialize. So double down on any meditations, affirmations, visualizations, journaling, or reading that will help you to imprint the desire to change your life. This is a powerful way to make it happen.

Also, join our private Facebook group at facebook.com/groups /DrKellyannsCleanseandReset/. You'll meet a fun and supportive community of people who'll be doing the cleanse right along with you.

3. Get your friends and family on board. Tell supportive people in your life what you're doing and why. Explain that you need to heal yourself, and that to do that you need to stick to the cleanse plan. Here's the speech I like to give:

"I'm doing a five-day cleanse because I'm not where I want to be, and I know that if I don't do anything, it's not going to get better—it's only going to get worse. I'm pretty confident about the track I'm on. Thank you in advance for being there for me and for not tempting me with foods that aren't on the plan."

If you're lucky, your friends and family will be so impressed with your plan that some will decide to do the cleanse with you! At a minimum, they'll know not to tempt you with "no" foods during your cleanse.

If you encounter people who aren't supportive, stay the course, because it's all about confidence. If they come at you like a pack of hyenas in *The Lion King*, don't let them in—because this is about you, and you're important.

4. Clean out your kitchen. The "no" foods on your cleanse—that is, any foods that aren't on the "yes" lists on pages 55 through 57—can't tempt you if they're not around. So toss out the foods you want to avoid, donate them to a food pantry, or ask a friend or neighbor to hold on to them until you finish the cleanse.

This goes for alcohol, too. After more than twenty years in practice, I know that alcohol is always the hardest thing for people to kiss goodbye for a few days. (Five minutes into a consult, I'm just waiting for each patient to say, "Don't tell me I can't have my glass of wine at night!") This is where you'll need to double down again on your resolve. Train your mind to pull up that TV screen showing your vision for your future.

If you can't get rid of "no" foods because other people in your home will be eating or drinking them, at least stick them toward the back of your pantry, fridge, or freezer. (Out of sight, out of mind.) Then dedicate a specific part of the refrigerator to your foods.

Also, if you're the family cook, consider making meals for your family members ahead of time and freezing them. That way, you won't be tempted to taste test during your cleanse. In addition, ask another person to do the serving and kitchen cleanup on your cleanse days.

For a printable list of "no" foods to clear out, visit the Resources page on my website at drkellyann.com/cleansebook.

5. Schedule a day to stock up and batch prep. After decades of guiding cleanses, I know that the biggest key to success is *preparation*. When your meals are right at your fingertips and ready to go every day, you won't be tempted to give in and grab the takeout menu when you're too tired to chop veggies or cook soup.

That's why I've planned this cleanse so you can do all of your shopping in a single trip to the store and then prep all of your meals in one or two easy sessions in the kitchen. In Chapter 4, right after I outline your cleanse, I'll tell you what to buy and how to make all of your meals in advance. So once you've picked the date when you'll begin your cleanse, schedule a shop-and-prep date just prior to Day 1.

By the way, batch prepping will be your friend even after your cleanse, because it makes eating healthy, fresh food *so* much easier. It's one of the best tricks I know to breaking the fast-food habit.

6. Make sure you have a source of clean water. When you're cleansing your body, you don't just want to give it clean food—you also want to give it clean water. And trust me: the water that comes out of your tap isn't clean. (I'll talk more about this in Chapter 6.) So if you don't currently have a water filtration system in your house, buy a water filtering pitcher at a minimum.

If you have a few extra dollars, also buy a water infuser bottle for making detox water. It's not necessary, but it's fun and handy.

7. Decide how you'll make or buy your smoothies. There are two options you can choose from when it comes to your smoothies, so pick one of these approaches:

- Buy a blender so you can make your own. This is by far your best option. If a good blender isn't in your budget, borrow one from a friend.

- Buy smoothie-bar smoothies if necessary—but be very, very careful! Most smoothies you'll get at a juice bar are way too high in sugar, so don't just order off the menu. Instead, get to be best friends with your baristas. Then tell them, "This is EXACTLY what I'd like in my drink," and give them your ingredient list. Also, make sure they're using water—not carrot, beet, or apple juice—as a base. As for grocery store smoothies, forget it; nearly all of them are packed with sugar.

8. Gently prepare your body. During the two to three days prior to starting your cleanse, drink lots of water to hydrate yourself. Ease off on heavy foods and carbs, and center your meals around lean proteins, leafy greens, and healthy fats. This will allow your body to transition easily to the cleanse.

9. Know what to expect day by day. Because I've guided lots of cleanses, I have a good feel for what you're going to experience on each day of your cleanse. While your results may vary a little, here's what I predict if you're doing the five days but not doing the Keto Push or staying on a keto plan for the entire cleanse (which I'll talk about below):

Day 1: This is your moment of exhilaration and excitement. You're still high energy and ready to roll.

Day 2: At this point, you're trying to get your groove down as you adapt to a different way of eating.

Day 3: You've got this down! You're noticing digestive changes for the better, and your bloat is disappearing.

Day 4: If you're limiting starchy veggies and fruits, you may feel a bit of the "carb flu" creeping about (more on this later, see page 43). Otherwise, you're feeling energized. You're also noticing that people are seeing a change in you, and you feel like your insides are cleaner.

Day 5: You love being squeaky-clean and may even think, "Is this thing over *already?*"

If you're doing the Keto Push and then following the standard cleanse, I'm betting that you'll get to the "squeaky-clean" stage even faster. (Yay!) That's because you'll already have one day under your belt when you start the cleanse itself. But you might need a little extra willpower toward the end of your cleanse since you've added that extra day up front. And you may be tempted by the "sugar demon" during your Keto Push (see page 48)—but stay strong!

If you do a keto version of the *entire* cleanse, in which you keep your carb count super-low, you'll want to be prepared for a few extra challenges you may encounter. That's because you're pushing your body to use stored fat for energy during your entire cleanse. In this case, you may get a longer visit from the sugar demon (see page 44), and the carb flu (see page 43) may strike as well. But remember that you're creating a super-efficient fat-burning system, so you'll get a big payoff in the end—especially if you're one of those people with that stubborn, stubborn belly fat.

Bothered by Bloat?

During your cleanse, you may experience a little temporary bloating as you change your gut's ecosystem for the better. If so, add these bloat-busting foods to your shakes, green smoothies, and soups:

Asparagus
Avocado
Cayenne pepper
Celery
Cucumbers
Fermented foods (sauerkraut, kimchi)
Ginger
Green tea
Lemon

10. Watch out for these two challenges! Okay, I'm not going to hold out on you. Instead, I'm going to warn you about two little antagonists that may pop up in this story. I call them the carb flu and the sugar demon, and the good news is that if you're ready for them, they won't slow you down at all. Here's what to do if they strike.

The Carb Flu

This is a very flexible cleanse, and it's your choice as to how many (if any) fruits and starchy veggies you'll include. If you're including them in most or all of your shakes, smoothies, and soups—which is what you'll do if you follow my recipes—you can skip this section. If not, read on.

If you choose to follow a keto version of this cleanse, and to minimize or eliminate fruits and starchy veggies (a good option if losing weight is a big goal for you), you're going to flip your fat-burning switch from "off" to "on." When you cut way down on carbs, your cells will start burning fat instead of sugar for fuel, rapidly melting away pounds of dangerous visceral fat.

This is a good thing—and if you're lucky, you'll blow through this transition effortlessly. However, there's a chance that you'll experience temporary symptoms I lovingly refer to as the "carb flu." The good news is that this icky stage goes away fast—and if you're ready for it, you'll breeze right through it.

Here's why the carb flu happens. Right now, if you're eating a diet that's high in carbs, your cells are in "easy" mode. You're constantly bathing them in sugar, so they don't have to work hard to get the fuel they need.

Burning fat is harder, and at first your cells won't like this at all. As a result, somewhere between Days 3 and 5, you may feel tired, cranky, wired, and weird. This isn't fun, but it's actually a great sign because it tells you that you're switching over to rapid fat-burning mode.

Here's a look at some of the symptoms you may experience when the carb flu sets in:

- You may feel tired. It's perfectly normal to run out of steam on carb flu days. If you can, keep your schedule light, and maybe even take a nap or go to bed early. A little coffee can help, but stick to just a few cups or you'll feel worse.

- You may feel "flu-ish." You might feel tired, develop "brain fog," or get a runny nose. But you're not really sick; it's just a temporary system overhaul.

- You may get moody. Your brain isn't happy right now because it's used to that heavy load of sugar and carbs. This moodiness, by the way, is related to your changing blood sugar levels. As you continue to eat real foods, you'll get your blood sugar under control and feel happy again.

- You may feel "icky." Digestive disturbances, allergies, and even outbreaks of acne may appear at this time. Remember that this is your body removing toxins and healing itself. At the end, you'll be rewarded with incredible energy, clear skin, glossy hair, a smaller waistline, and glowing health.

The key to getting through the carb flu is to know why it's happening and understand that it's temporary. Once you're past it, your body will burn fat effortlessly, and you'll feel renewed and revitalized.

In the meantime, here are some strategies that can make the carb flu easier on you:

- Journal every day. This will help you spot the signs of the carb flu and recognize it for what it is.
- Do a little light exercise—for instance, take a walk.
- Do the cleanse with a friend if you can. That way, you can give each other moral support if the carb flu strikes.

The Sugar Demon

The sugar demon and you . . . have you met?

If you're a sugar freak, you know what I'm talking about, and I won't lie—limiting your sugar for five days will challenge you if you're used to a steady stream of sweet treats and sodas. That's because you're genetically wired to crave that sugar.

You see, back when we lived in caves, having a sweet tooth used to be pro-survival. Sugar was scarce then, it provided energy for people who burned lots of fuel hunting and gathering, and it came packaged in healthy foods like berries and honey.

In other words, sugar worked for us back then, so Mother Nature wired us to love it and seek it out.

Now, however, sugar is everywhere, and it's packaged in all kinds of junk food that makes us fat and sick. Worse yet, manufacturers now load products with tons of high-fructose corn syrup, which is even worse for us.

Even though we know these foods are bad for us, we still crave them. In fact, *crave* might be too mild a word because research shows that many of us are actually addicted to sugar. In an eye-opening 2018 study, researchers asked soda-guzzling teens to refrain from drinking sugar-sweetened drinks for three days. Participants reported withdrawal symptoms including cravings, headaches, reduced well-being, impaired concentration, and decreased motivation to work.[1] In an earlier study, rats allowed to choose between cocaine and Oreos went for the Oreos as often as the cocaine.[2]

Clearly, sugar can sink its claws deep into you. So how do you break the sugar demon's hold? While it's tough at first, the best solution is to go cold turkey and cut sugar completely out of your diet. In fact, if you ask me to name the most important thing you can do—just *one thing* that's best for your health and to protect against aging—I'll tell you that it's swearing off all forms of sugar. And believe it or not, when you do this, you'll eventually stop craving sweets.

Right now, however, I just need you to limit yourself to healthy sugars from fruit and starchy veggies for a few days and cut out all the rest. (You can do that, right?) Of course, if you're doing a keto modification of the cleanse and cutting out even these healthy foods, you'll have a bigger challenge. Just remember that you're getting a bigger payoff as well: that extra belly fat you'll be blasting.

To help you resist the siren song of cookies, candy, and soda, remember that the average craving lasts only three minutes. Distract yourself by playing a game on your phone, taking a walk, or calling a friend—and before you know it, that craving will be history.

Finally, remember what I said earlier: when you commit to a life-changing project, keep the end in mind. Think about how you got where you are now, and where you want to go. Keep your mind on how happy, slim, restored, and rejuvenated you'll be at the end of your cleanse. That's sweeter than a sugary treat, right?

Have a Sweet Tooth? Try Monk Fruit!

On this cleanse, you can add either stevia or monk fruit to your shakes and green smoothies if you like. Odds are, you've already tried stevia, since it's been on the market for ages—but is monk fruit new to you?

If so, here's the story. Monk fruit is a Chinese fruit known as *luo han guo*. It looks a little like a green lemon, but it's hiding a sweet secret: its pulp is 300 times sweeter than sugar. When it's turned into a liquid or powdered sweetener, you get a big burst of sweetness for close to zero calories.

Monk fruit has been used as a sweetener and herbal medicine for centuries in Asian countries, and now it's catching on in the West. That's a good trend because monk fruit has some amazing health benefits. It contains antioxidants called *mogrosides* that pack a powerful punch, helping to protect you against everything from cancer to diabetes and its complications. Here's a sampling of the research:

• One study reported that a mogroside extract lowered blood sugar levels, oxidative stress, and lipid levels in diabetic mice, suggesting that it could help prevent diabetic complications in humans.[3]

- Mogrosides can help you slim down. Both a 2018 study[4] and a 2012 study[5] found that they protected against obesity in mice eating an unhealthy diet.
- A study of mice with gestational diabetes, a type of diabetes that develops during pregnancy, found that giving them one type of mogroside found in monk fruit improved glucose metabolism, reduced insulin resistance, and led to healthier offspring.[6]
- A study published in 2016 found that one type of mogrosides, mogroside V, suppressed the growth of tumors in pancreatic cancer.[7] Other research shows that mogrosides may help fight colorectal and throat cancer.[8]

And unlike artificial sweeteners, monk fruit has no known adverse side effects. In fact, research indicates that even in super-high doses, it's safe.[9]

In short, monk fruit appears to be all upside and no downside—so if the sugar demon is getting you down and you're really craving some sweetness, I highly recommend giving it a try.

You're Ready to Go!

At this point, you're fully on track for success. You're ready both physically and emotionally for this big moment in your life. You have your goals firmly in mind, you have your friends and family on board, and you know how to keep the carb flu and the sugar demon from sabotaging your plan.

There's no stopping you now . . . so it's time to jump into your cleanse!

Chapter 4

Doing Your Cleanse

know you're happy that you've decided to splurge on yourself and go for this cleanse. What I've come to realize—and maybe you have too—is that *health and beauty really are the new luxury.*

So let's go get them!

In this chapter, I'll fill you in on all the details about your cleanse, including how to shop and prep for it in advance. Once you're up to speed, you'll be fully prepared to head for the starting line.

Your One-Day "Keto Push" (Optional)

Reminder: This is NOT part of your five-day cleanse! Think of it as a Day Zero pre-cleanse. If you prefer not to do it, simply skip this section and go to the next one. It's totally up to you.

If you're opting to do the Keto Push, I want you to spend twenty-four hours drinking water or bone broth. (You can also have unsweetened coffee or tea—no creamer or artificial sweeteners.) This will push your body into rapid fat-burning, especially around your belly. As a result, you'll be ahead of the game before you even start your cleanse!

Your Cleanse Plan, Step-by-Step

If you're skipping the Keto Push, this is where you'll start. If not, this is where you'll start *after* your one-day Keto Push.

Note: If you want to stay in ketosis for the entire cleanse, see page 52 for instructions and recipes.

You're going to love how easy this cleanse is, especially if you've done your up-front shake and smoothie prep (see page 53) and you've made your broth loading soups. It's as simple as heating broth and pushing buttons on your blender. (Oh, and slicing a lemon each day.) I would never ask you to do something I wouldn't do myself, so you can trust that this is going to be painless.

Over the next five days, you're going to load your body with nutrients and cleanse it of toxins by rotating green smoothies, collagen shakes, and nourishing soups. Here's what you'll do each day:

1. Start your morning with refreshing lemon water. Each morning, I want you to drink a glass of hot or cold lemon water, adding a few fresh herbs like basil or mint. This will give you a good dose of vitamin C—a nutrient that's crucial for building that gut-healing, skin-firming collagen. Also, those herbs are powerhouses of healing nutrients—I'll talk about this in a little bit (see page 60).

To make your lemon water, muddle your herbs first with a wooden spoon or muddler, and then add water and the juice of half a lemon.

Oh, and you can also have coffee in the morning (and at any other time you want it). I want you to know this upfront because otherwise this would be the Five-Minute Cleanse, and you'd close the book right now.

2. Have a green smoothie for breakfast. Your first meal of the day will be a green smoothie loaded with what I call "high-vibe" nutrients to make your cellular matrix sparkle. This will give you a big blast of energy.

Each of your smoothies will contain:

1. One to two scoops of collagen or bone broth protein powder
2. A healthy fat from the list on page 57

3. A fruit or starchy veggie from the list on pages 55 and 56 (unless you're doing the keto modification)
4. Two handfuls of non-starchy veggies
5. Stevia or monk fruit, if desired
6. Herbs and spices, if desired

In Chapter 7, you'll find lots of recipes for yummy green smoothies featuring all of your favorite ingredients.

Note: This is a good time to take a multivitamin and multimineral supplement (if you're taking one—if not, see my note on page 15 about foods you'll want to add to your cleanse). However, you can take it with any meal.

3. Have a collagen shake for lunch. Here, you'll get another hefty dose of that beautiful collagen. Each of your shakes will contain:

1. One to two scoops of collagen or bone broth protein powder
2. One cup of unsweetened almond milk or coconut milk (not canned) or water
3. A healthy fat from the list on page 57
4. One serving of fruit or starchy veggies, if desired (unless you're doing the keto modification)
5. Two handfuls of leafy greens (optional)
6. Stevia or monk fruit, if desired
7. Herbs and spices, if desired

In Chapter 8, you'll find recipes for shakes that feature all of your favorite flavors, from piña colada to chocolate raspberry and peachy almond. Who says a cleanse can't be delicious? If you're feeling creative, you can come up with your own recipes—just be sure to stick to the guidelines above.

4. Have another green smoothie around midafternoon. Now it's time to reload your body with those fabulous plant nutrients, along with another serving of collagen. Follow the same guidelines as you did in the morning, building your smoothie from these ingredients:

1. One to two scoops of collagen or bone broth protein powder
2. A healthy fat from the list on page 57
3. A fruit or starchy veggie from the list on pages 55 and 56 (unless you're doing the keto modification)
4. Two handfuls of non-starchy veggies
5. Stevia or monk fruit, if desired
6. Herbs and spices if, desired

5. Have a rich, delicious broth loading soup for dinner. At the end of your day, you'll relax with a warm, satisfying soup loaded with more cleansing, revitalizing veggies. Your soup will contain:

1. One to two cups of broth
2. One serving of a healthy fat, such as full-fat coconut milk or avocado
3. Lots of non-starchy veggies (load up on them!)
4. One (optional) serving of a starchy veggie (unless you're doing the keto modification)
5. Herbs and spices, if desired

You'll find lots of absolutely delicious soup recipes in Chapter 9, and feel free to invent your own as well—all you have to do is reference the ingredient list above.

6. Any time you want, you can have these "freebies." Unsweetened coffee and tea are on the unlimited list. You can also keep your body purring with clean, cool detox water (you'll find fun recipes in Chapter 10).

Doing Keto for Your Entire Cleanse?

After your "Keto Push," you can opt to follow a keto modification of this entire cleanse. If you do, simply eliminate fruits (except for small amounts of berries or grapefruit) and stick to non-starchy veggies. Here is a list of the recipes in this book that are keto-friendly.

Green Smoothies
- Lemon Ginger Green Smoothie (page 147)
- Mexican Fiesta Green Smoothie (page 148)
- Savory Mediterranean Green Smoothie (page 151)
- Savory Salad Bowl Smoothie (page 152)

Shakes
- Lemon Cream Shake (page 167)
- Chocolate Raspberry Shake (page 171)
- Other shake recipes, if you eliminate the fruit and starchy veggies

Broth Loading Soups
- Creamy Asparagus Soup (page 191)
- Roasted Curried Cauliflower Soup (page 194)
- Thai Red Curry Soup (page 199)
- Tom Kha Gai (page 201)
- Chilled Cucumber Soup (page 203)
- Creamy Broccoli Soup (page 204)
- Watercress Soup (page 205)
- Cauliflower Vichyssoise (page 206)

How to Shop and Prep for Your Cleanse

When you do all of your shopping and batch prep *before* you start your cleanse, your meals will be a breeze. You'll have your shakes, green smoothies, and soups ready in seconds—no fuss and no stress. Here's how to do it:

First, plan your shopping trip. Flip through the recipes in Chapters 7 through 10, decide which ones you want to make, and make a list of the ingredients. (If you want a quick and easy alternative, use my five-day meal plan and shopping list on pages 58 through 60 instead.) This way, you can buy all of your ingredients in a single trip. (Remember to add in a multivitamin and multimineral supplement if you're using one; if not, see my tips on page 15.)

One note: when you're buying your collagen or protein powder, select a high-quality brand made from pastured beef. (Dr. Kellyann's Collagen Shake, Dr. Kellyann's Bone Broth Protein, and Dr. Kellyann's Flavorless Collagen Protein for green smoothies are great choices.) Be sure to look for the word *beef* on the label. Don't settle for whey protein powder because many people are allergic to whey. And don't use pea powder either, unless you're doing my vegetarian or vegan modification, because it's higher in carbs and isn't as nutrient-dense.

One serving of protein or collagen powder is equal to one to two scoops of powder. Plan to have 10 to 25 grams of protein in each shake or green smoothie.

A Quick Look at Coconut Milk

Many of my broth loading soup recipes and shake recipes call for uncanned or canned coconut milk. If you're new to coconut milk, here's a quick primer so you'll know that you're buying the right type of coconut milk—and so you'll understand why some recipes call for two different types of coconut milk!

Coconut Milk (not canned)—Your "Base" Liquid

This is a thin liquid—you'll find it in the refrigerated case at the store along with other milks, or in unrefrigerated cartons—that contains very little fat. It doesn't count as a fat on your cleanse, so you can use it as the liquid base for your shakes. If you buy this type of coconut milk, make sure it's free of added sugars and carrageenan, an additive that's highly inflammatory (see page 168).

Coconut Milk in a Can—For a Dose of Healthy Fat

Canned coconut milk has much the same consistency as whipping cream. It's an ingredient in several of the soups, and you can also add ⅓ cup to shakes (do count it as a fat). That's why some shakes have two types of coconut milk: non-canned coconut milk as a base and canned coconut milk as a fat.

When you're buying canned coconut milk, always choose full-fat rather than low-fat; it tastes better, and it's better for you. In addition, try to find a brand in a BPA-free can.

Canned coconut milk typically separates in the can, creating a thick layer of cream on top and a thinner layer of milk on the bottom. That's why it's a good idea to shake the can vigorously before you open it.

Next, make your bone broth (unless you're buying it). You'll need at least two-and-a-half quarts of bone broth (about 80 ounces) for your five days. You'll find easy recipes in Chapter 9, and you can make all the broth you need for your cleanse in a single afternoon. (It can simmer happily on the stove while you're chopping your veggies.)

Once you've made your broth, you can select the soups you want to make with it. All of these soups freeze beautifully, so you can make them in advance. If you can swing it, buy an immersion blender; it's a handy way to blend your "cream" soups. If not, you can blend them in a blender or food processor.

Finally, prep your fruits and veggies for your smoothies and shakes. Wash them, chop them, and freeze them in individual servings, so they'll be ready to grab and toss into your blender. You can also toss in any herbs and spices the recipes call for.

Your "Yes" Veggies, Fruits, and Fats

All of the recipes in this book are designed specifically for your cleanse. But if you love making up your own recipes, go for it!

Here are the veggies, fruits, and fats you can choose from. To keep your carb count for the day to around 60 carbs, you'll want to limit each meal to about 15 carbs. If you want specific carb counts for each fruit and veggie, see pages 232 through 237; otherwise, simply follow the guidelines in the chart.

"Yes" Fruits and Vegetables for Your Cleanse

UNLIMITED	LIMITED (one serving per meal)—avoid if you are doing the keto modification
Leafy greens and non-starchy veggies:	Starchy veggies (half a cup):
Arugula	Acorn squash
Asparagus	Beets
Bell peppers	Butternut squash
Bok choy	Carrots
Broccoli	Celery root
Broccoli rabe	Jicama
Brussels sprouts	Kohlrabi
Cauliflower	Parsnips
Celery	Plantains
Chile peppers	Pumpkin
Cilantro	Rutabaga
Cucumbers	Spaghetti squash
Daikon	Sweet potatoes and yams

UNLIMITED	LIMITED (one serving per meal)—avoid if you are doing the keto modification
Leafy greens and non-starchy veggies:	*Starchy veggies (half a cup):*
Eggplant	Turnips
Garlic	Yucca
Green beans	*Fruits (half a cup):*
Green cabbage	Apple
Green onions	Apricot
Greens (beet, collard, mustard, and turnip greens)	Blackberries
Jalapeño peppers	Blueberries
Kale	Boysenberry
Leeks	Cantaloupe
Lettuce	Cherry
Mushrooms	Clementine
Napa cabbage	Cranberry
Onions	Grapefruit
Parsley	Guava
Radicchio	Honeydew
Radishes	Kiwi
Red cabbage	Lemon
Seaweed	Lime
Spinach	Mango
Sprouts	Mulberry
Summer squash	Nectarine
Swiss chard	Orange
Tomato	Papaya
Watercress	Peach
Zucchini	Pear
	Pineapple
	Plum
	Raspberries
	Star fruit
	Strawberries
	Tangerine
	Watermelon

"Yes" Fats for Your Cleanse

Almond butter	unsweetened; 1 tablespoon per serving
Avocado	1/4 to 1/2 avocado per serving
Avocado oil	1 tablespoon per serving
Canned full-fat coconut milk	1/3 cup
Chia seeds	4 teaspoons per serving
Coconut chips	unsweetened; 1 closed handful or about 2 tablespoons per serving
Coconut oil / MCT oil	1 tablespoon per serving
Ghee (clarified butter—see below)	1 tablespoon per serving
Ground flaxseed	2 tablespoons per serving
Hemp seeds	2 tablespoons per serving
Nuts	1 closed handful per serving, about 2 tablespoons; don't use peanuts or peanut butter
Olive oil	1 tablespoon per serving
Olives	1 closed handful per serving or about 2 tablespoons
Walnut oil	1 tablespoon per serving

How to Make Ghee

You can buy ghee, or clarified butter, in many health food stores. However, it's also a cinch to make it at home. Simply heat a stick of butter gently, then skim off the milk solids with a mesh strainer when they come to the top. Cool the ghee and keep it refrigerated.

Sample Meal Plan

If you'd like to make planning your meals super-easy, just follow this five-day meal plan and buy the ingredients listed in the shopping list that follows it. It can't get simpler than that! (For a printable meal plan, visit my Resources page at drkellyann.com/cleansebook.)

DAY	GREEN SMOOTHIE	SHAKE	GREEN SMOOTHIE	SOUP
1	Pineapple Mint Green Smoothie	Chocolate Raspberry Shake	Strawberry Green Smoothie	Chicken and "Rice" Soup
2	Cucumber Melon Green Smoothie	Piña Colada Shake	Lemon Ginger Green Smoothie	Creamy Asparagus Soup
3	Papaya Ginger Green Smoothie	Chocolate Raspberry Shake	Pineapple Mint Green Smoothie	Chicken and "Rice" Soup
4	Strawberry Green Smoothie	Apple Pie Shake	Cucumber Melon Green Smoothie	Creamy Asparagus Soup
5	Lemon Ginger Green Smoothie	Piña Colada Shake	Papaya Ginger Green Smoothie	Chicken and "Rice" Soup

Shopping List for Sample Five-Day Meal Plan

Here are all the groceries you'll need to buy to make everything in this meal plan. (For a printable shopping list and a list of recommended brands, visit the Resources page on my website at drkellyann.com/cleansebook.)

PRODUCE
Apple (1 small)
Asparagus (1 pound)
Carrots (1 pound)
Cauliflower (1 medium head)
Celery (1 bunch)

Cucumbers (1, English preferred)
Garlic (1 head)
Ginger root (4- to 5-inch knob)
Honeydew melon (1 medium)
Kale (1 large bunch, to yield 4 cups chopped)
Leeks (2)
Lemons (3)
Mint (1 bunch, fresh)
Onion (1 small)
Papaya (1 large)
Parsley (1 bunch)
Pineapple (1 large fresh or 1 bag frozen, to yield 3 cups)
Limes (2)
Raspberries (1 small box, to yield 1 cup)
Romaine lettuce (1 head)
Spinach (5-ounce box of fresh baby spinach, to yield 4 cups)
Strawberries (1 pint)
Thyme (1 small bunch, or dried)

REFRIGERATED
Coconut or almond milk (½ gallon)
Ghee or pasture-raised butter (¼ pound)

GROCERY
Arrowroot (smallest size)
Avocado oil or olive oil (smallest bottle)
Black pepper
Canned full-fat coconut milk (five 14-ounce cans)
Celtic or pink Himalayan salt
Chia seeds (small bag)
Chocolate collagen protein—5 servings, 15 to 25 grams protein per
    serving
Cinnamon

Nutmeg

Stevia or monk fruit sweetener

Flavorless collagen—5 servings, 15 to 25 grams protein per serving

Vanilla collagen protein—5 servings, 15 to 25 grams protein per serving

BONE BROTH

Chicken bone broth (½ gallon or 8 cups)

If you are making your own chicken bone broth, you will need the following ingredients. All other ingredients you need are already on the shopping list:

2 or more pounds chicken thighs, legs, and/or wings

3 or more pounds raw or cooked chicken bones/carcasses

6 to 8 chicken feet, optional, but will add a great deal of collagen to your broth

Apple cider vinegar

Bay leaf (optional)

Onion (1 medium)

Peppercorns (or substitute black pepper)

ADDITIONAL

Multivitamin and multimineral supplement (if you are using one)

Detox water ingredients (if you plan to make any)

Spice It Up!

Want to add even more cleaning, healing, and fat-burning power to your cleanse? Then toss some of the following herbs and spices into your bone broth, shakes, and green smoothies. Here's why they're so awesome:

- **Basil.** Basil is anti-inflammatory, reduces water retention and bloating, and is an *adaptogen* (a substance that helps your body adapt to stress). Basil also helps reduce fat buildup in your liver while detoxifying your body. Even the scent of basil is known to have healing properties.

- **Black pepper.** *Piperine* is the compound that gives pepper its pungent flavor. Piperine enhances the effects of curcumin, the active ingredient in turmeric—a fat-burning spice I'll talk about later. One study also suggests that the piperine in black pepper battles fat by blocking the formation of new fat cells.[1]

- **Cardamom.** Cardamom is *thermogenic* (meaning it increases your body heat and speeds up your metabolism), has anti-inflammatory properties, and acts as an antioxidant, cleaning up rogue molecules called free radicals and resisting cellular aging.

- **Cayenne.** This is my personal favorite. There's no better natural fat-burner, which is why I put it in just about everything I can get my hands on. *Capsaicin*, the compound that gives chile peppers their heat, helps shrink fatty tissue and lower blood-fat levels. It's also thermogenic.

- **Cilantro and coriander.** Although both names refer to the same plant, *cilantro* typically refers to the leafy green part of the coriander plant, while *coriander* is the common name for the seeds of the plant. Both cilantro and coriander are antioxidant-rich and may help reduce LDL, or "bad," cholesterol levels in your blood. They also contain large quantities of vitamins A and K. And let's face it: everything tastes better with cilantro.

- **Cinnamon.** Cinnamon is a spice worth taking seriously at a time when blood sugar problems are pandemic. It's so simple, yet it can dramatically lower your blood glucose. It can also reduce your cravings and help you burn fat faster.

- **Cloves.** Cloves help reduce your blood sugar. They also help improve your digestion and optimize your metabolism.

- **Cumin.** Cumin is a great fat burner that also aids in digestion. One teaspoon can help you burn up to *three times* more body fat.
- **Fennel seeds.** These are a natural diuretic and an effective digestive aid.
- **Garlic.** Garlic helps burn belly fat. It also reduces LDL cholesterol, which may lower your risk of heart disease. In addition, it reduces oxidative damage from free radicals, helping fight the aging process.
- **Ginger.** Ginger has anti-inflammatory properties, and it's a great gut soother. It also has thermogenic properties that help boost your metabolism.
- **Green and white teas.** These teas are loaded with antioxidants and thermogenic properties. What's more, they contain a compound called epigallocatechin gallate (EGCG) that reduces the amount of fat your body absorbs when you eat.
- **Mustard.** One teaspoon of prepared mustard can boost your metabolism by up to 25% for several hours after eating. This effect is due to allyl isothiocyanates, which are phytochemicals that give mustard its characteristic flavor.
- **Parsley.** Parsley's wealth of vitamin C makes it a great immune-system booster. It's also an excellent source of beta-carotene, an antioxidant that helps protect your body against free-radical damage. It has anti-inflammatory properties, relaxes your muscles, and encourages digestion.
- **Turmeric.** Curcumin is the active ingredient in turmeric. It slows the formation of fatty tissue by affecting the blood vessels needed to form it. Curcumin contributes to lower body fat and weight loss. It is also an anti-inflammatory agent and lowers insulin resistance.
- **White pepper.** As with black pepper, piperine is the compound that gives white pepper its pungent flavor. Like black pepper, white pepper increases the effects of curcumin, the active ingredient in turmeric.

Add Green Tea for More Detox Power

Green tea is delicious, and it can add extra octane to your cleanse. Here are some of its benefits:

- It helps to clean toxins out of your system. Research shows that green tea dramatically boosts your body's production of a type of enzymes called GST enzymes, which play a key role in defending your body against cancer-causing chemicals and other toxins.[2]
- It's loaded with powerful cell-protecting antioxidants called *catechins*, and it has about eight to ten times more polyphenols than fruits and vegetables.[3]
- It helps to slim you down. Green tea increases thermogenesis (heat production), helping you burn off fat more quickly. According to a recent review, long-term studies show that "the consumption of tea catechins induces a notable reduction of body weight and body fat."[4]

One caution, however: concentrated forms of green tea (such as green tea extract) might be dangerous. In some cases, people using these concentrated forms have suffered liver damage.

So here's my advice: skip the extract, and get the benefits of green tea the old-fashioned way—by brewing up a nice, warm mug of it. To get the most benefit, use boiling water (which helps release the antioxidants in the tea) and let the tea steep for two to five minutes.

Add More Collagen Boosters

You can take your collagen-building to the next level by adding lots of collagen "buddies"—foods that promote collagen formation or prevent its breakdown—to your shakes, green smoothies, and soups. Here are three ways to boost your collagen production during and after your cleanse:

1. **Load up on foods high in vitamin C.** Vitamin C is vital for the synthesis of collagen. It's a limiting factor, meaning that if you don't have enough, your collagen production line shuts down. So eat plenty of foods rich in vitamin C, including tomatoes, bell peppers, and broccoli.

2. **Eat different colors of veggies.** Dark, leafy greens like spinach and kale contain antioxidants that protect against the free radicals that break down collagen. Red veggies like beets (as well as fruits like tomatoes and red peppers) are full of lycopene, which boosts collagen and protects against sun damage. And orange veggies like carrots and sweet potatoes are loaded with vitamin A, which restores collagen that's been damaged.

3. **Drink unsweetened white tea.** White tea is light and delicate, but it packs a big punch when it comes to fighting wrinkles. Research shows that it helps to thwart the activities of enzymes that break down collagen and another skin protein, elastin.

When You're Done with Your Cleanse, Ease Back into Eating

When you're finished with your cleanse, I want you to eat lightly for two to three days before getting back to your usual diet. I recommend eating small servings of clean, natural, easy-to-digest foods—for instance, lean poultry or fish, sautéed veggies, and berries—and then slowly adding in other foods over time.

If you're not at your goal weight at the end of this time, you can transition directly to my 21-Day Bone Broth Diet or my 10-Day Belly Slimdown. If you have reached your goal weight, move on to Dr. Kellyann's Lifestyle Plan (see Chapter 11), which will allow you to maintain your cleanse wins.

More Great Cleanse Teas

Three more teas that can boost the effects of your cleanse are milk thistle, dandelion, and burdock teas. Here's a look at each one:

- Milk thistle tea, made from crushed seeds from the milk thistle plant (*Silybum marianum*), is a powerful liver healer. Silymarin, a compound in milk thistle, has antioxidant, anti-inflammatory, and antiviral properties—and it may help to keep you looking young by protecting your skin against sun damage.[5]
- Dandelion tea is another powerful liver healer and if you need quick relief from bloating, it's a diuretic that can flush out extra water. In addition, it has anti-diabetic properties.
- Burdock tea is prized by many cultures as a blood purifier, and science shows that it has liver-protective and detoxifying properties.[6]

One note: avoid dandelion, milk thistle, and burdock teas if you're allergic to ragweed, marigolds, chrysanthemums, and related plants. If you have any plant allergies at all, test a small amount first to make sure you do fine with it.

A Word About Cheats

Sometimes, even when you have the best of intentions, life can get in the way. For instance, there's a chance that you'll start this cleanse strong and then get derailed partway through by a family crisis, a breakup, or some other calamity.

If that happens, it's perfectly okay—so don't beat yourself up over it. Instead, count each cleanse day you finished as a big win and schedule another cleanse for the near future. Remember: your bone broth and the fruits and veggies you've prepped will wait patiently for you in the freezer!

How About Coffee?

Good news: I love coffee, and I'm a firm believer that it adds power to a cleanse. That's why it's a big "yes" on this plan.

It's a common belief that coffee pulls water out of your body, and for this reason coffee is often a big no-no on other cleanse protocols. But as it turns out, this is a myth. One study asked coffee drinkers to consume either coffee or water for three days, and the researchers found no difference between the hydration status of the two groups.[7]

So go ahead and count coffee as part of your water intake each day. In fact, I encourage it because coffee has so many health benefits. Here are just some of them:

- Drinking three or four cups of coffee each day appears to lower your risk of diabetes.[8]
- Caffeinated coffee consumption may help to protect you against dementia.[9]
- Coffee may even help you live longer. One study analyzed coffee consumption over an average of more than sixteen

years among more than 185,000 people. The researchers found that drinking one cup of coffee a day was linked to a 12% lower risk of death at any age, from any cause. People drinking two or three cups a day had an 18% lower risk.[10]

What's more, caffeinated coffee is *ergogenic*—that is, it enhances your performance when you work out and keeps you burning more calories long afterward. Here's a sampling of the findings:

- Athletes burned 15% more calories after a cycling workout when they took a dose of caffeine before their workouts instead of a placebo.[11]
- Stationary bike riders burned more calories when they consumed caffeine before exercising, compared to when they took a placebo—and they also enjoyed exercising more.[12]
- Weightlifters did more repetitions after getting a dose of caffeine, and the caffeine reduced their feelings of exertion and pain.[13]

So caffeine helps you stay diabetes-free, protects you from dementia, helps you burn more fat, and eases workout-related aches and pains. What's not to love about that?

Modifying the Cleanse for Special Diets

Lots of my patients follow vegan, vegetarian or, pescatarian diets. If you belong to any of these groups, don't worry—I've got you covered! Here's how to modify the cleanse to suit any type of diet.

How to Do This Cleanse If You're a Vegetarian or Vegan

If your diet doesn't include animal products such as collagen or bone broth, you might be wondering: How can you do a cleanse that features collagen *without* eating collagen? Luckily, it's easier than it sounds. Here's how to modify the cleanse to work for you:

- Replace the bone broth with vegetable broth (see recipe on page 185). (An aside: while I love bone broth, I'm also a big fan of veggie broth—often called potassium broth because it's loaded with this nutrient. In particular, I drink veggie broth if I'm having problems with cramps.)
- Omit the collagen powder from your green smoothies.
- Use egg, pea, or hemp powder in place of collagen powder in your shakes.

While your cleanse won't include actual collagen, it will include *building blocks* of collagen. When you build your broth loading soups, green smoothies, and shakes, focus in particular on foods that are high in glycine and proline, the primary amino acids in collagen. Select lots of these fruits and veggies.

BEST SOURCES OF GLYCINE

- Banana
- Cabbage
- Cauliflower
- Cucumber
- Kale
- Kiwi
- Pumpkin
- Spinach

BEST SOURCES OF PROLINE
- Alfalfa sprouts
- Asparagus
- Cabbage
- Chives
- Cucumber
- Watercress
- White mustard seeds

Also, add foods rich in the amino acid lysine to your shakes and green smoothies. These include pistachios and pumpkin seeds.

Finally, incorporate lots of "collagen buddies" into your meals (see the list of them on page 64). These are foods that your body needs to synthesize new collagen and protect your existing stores.

How to Do This Cleanse If You're a Pescatarian

If you limit your intake of animal products to fish and seafood, you can make a beautiful fish bone broth to use in your broth loading soups. (See the Seafood Bone Broth recipe on page 183.) For your shakes and green smoothies, substitute marine collagen for beef collagen.

Cleanse FAQs

Here are some of the most common questions I get about my cleanse.

Is this cleanse considered keto, paleo, or low-carb?
It works with all three diets. That's because it's low in carbs, all of the foods on the plan are paleo-compliant, and if you cut out the fruits and starchy veggies, it will keep you in ketosis.

Should I weigh myself every day on this cleanse?

I know you want to, and I don't want to be a meanie, but no—resist the urge to hop on the scale every morning. You need to allow your body to readjust and repopulate your flora, and this takes time. This is not a moment when you need to hang on to metrics. You have to trust your body and let it do what it's designed to do.

How often can I do this cleanse?

You can do it as often as monthly, and I recommend doing it at least once every three or four months. Making it a regular habit is a smart way to sustain weight loss and to make sure you're always at your best.

Can I take my regular vitamins and probiotics?

Yes. You can keep taking any supplements you're currently using. Just be sure to take them with a meal rather than on an empty stomach.

Can I take my medication?

Check with your doctor to make sure you can do this cleanse while taking your current medications. Also, ask if you will need to change your dosage. (This is especially important if you're taking drugs for diabetes or metabolic syndrome.) If you get a thumbs-up from your doctor, you're good to go.

Can I have kombucha?

Okay, don't hate me here. I want you to avoid kombucha on your cleanse because not all kombucha drinks are alike and some have enough sugar to derail your cleanse. So for now, put kombucha on your "no" list. After your cleanse, it's fine on Dr. Kellyann's Lifestyle Plan—the "forever" plan you'll start on after you finish your cleanse and you've reached your goal weight.

Can I add monk fruit, stevia, collagen, coconut oil, or cream to my coffee?

Monk fruit and stevia are a "yes." (See page 46 for info on why monk fruit is so good for you.) However, I want you to avoid adding collagen or coconut oil to your coffee because you'll get plenty of collagen and healthy fats in your meals, and that's where you need them to help you absorb and metabolize all the phytonutrients you're getting. So promise me you won't "steal" collagen or fats from your meals to use in your coffee! Also, avoid cream and any artificial sweeteners or creamers.

Can I use powdered greens or powdered superfood in my green smoothies?

Fresh is best because a powder can't provide all of the fiber that fresh greens give you. However, it's fine to get your greens in powdered form if the convenience factor is important for you. Just check the label and make sure the powder doesn't contain sugar, artificial sweeteners, artificial colors or flavors, or emulsifiers. For recommended brands of powdered greens, please visit the Resources page on my website at drkellyann.com/cleansebook.

Can I eat foods that aren't on the "yes" list?

I've selected the "yes" foods to give you the best results. Stay strong, stick to the foods on the "yes" list, and you'll love the results you get!

Can I chew gum on this diet?

I don't recommend it because it confuses your body and makes your digestive system think that solid food is coming. Also, most gum is loaded with artificial flavors and colors. Once you're done with your cleanse, a healthy, additive-free type of gum (such as Spry) is fine when you've moved on to Dr. Kellyann's Lifestyle Plan (you'll learn more about this phase in Chapter 5).

Can I exercise, or should I pause my exercise routine?
This is entirely up to you. Some people can easily do heavy gym work-outs during their cleanse, while others find strenuous exercise too hard. If you're in the second group, it's a good idea to lighten up on your workouts or even skip them, so your body can invest all of its energy in healing. Once you finish your cleanse, you'll have so much energy that you'll more than make up for lost workout time!

Can I have your collagen products on my cleanse?
Absolutely. They're all designed to be compliant with this cleanse as well as my Bone Broth Diet and 10-Day Belly Slimdown.

Do I have to do five days? Can I do less? Can I do more?
Even one or two days on this cleanse will make you feel better. How-ever, it takes five days to get the full benefits, so do the full cleanse if you can. If you feel like you want even more healing power, do the Keto Push up front or add an extra day or two at the end of the cleanse—or consider switching over to my Bone Broth Diet or 10-Day Belly Slimdown.

Can I eat any fats on this cleanse?
You'll eat fats every day, but make sure you eat the right ones (see my list on page 57). I want you to avoid margarine and inflammatory seed oils like corn, sunflower, safflower, and canola oil.

Can I drink sparkling water while I'm doing the cleanse?
Yes, but be aware that sparkling water can cause you to bloat. Drink just a little at a time and be sure to choose plain sparkling water rather than water with added flavors or colors.

What's really important is to get plenty of water—whether it's spar-kling or not. This is a big key to flushing out toxins.

Why can't I use artificial sweeteners on this cleanse?
I know this is a toughie for many people, especially if they're used to drinking diet sodas all day. But the fact is those artificial sweeteners can actually be worse for you than sugar.

In a 2018 study, researchers tested six artificial sweeteners—aspartame, sucralose, neotame, saccharine, advantame, and acesulfame potassium—and found that the sweeteners caused gut bacteria in mice to become toxic.[14] That's the last thing you want on a cleanse!

I see something called MCT oil on the list of good fats. What is that?
MCT stands for *medium-chain triglyceride.* MCTs are the cleanest, most direct sources of energy for your body. Your body metabolizes these fatty acids in a different way than it does other fatty acids, increasing the number of calories you burn.

Because they're rapidly turned into ketones, MCTs also give your brain a quick shot of energizing fuel. In addition, studies show that they're an excellent weight-loss tool. For instance:

- In a sixteen-week trial, thirty-one overweight men and women in a weight-loss program consumed either olive oil or MCT oil in their diets. The researchers found that the MCT oil group lost more weight, more fat mass overall, and more trunk mass than the olive-oil group.[15]
- In another study, twenty-four healthy overweight men ate diets rich in either MCT oil or olive oil for twenty-eight days and then switched over. The researchers found that participants lost more weight in the MCT oil phase and concluded, "MCTs may be considered as agents that aid in the prevention of obesity or potentially stimulate weight loss."[16]

So add a serving of them to your broth, shakes, or green smoothies, and you'll take your fat burning to an even higher level. One caution:

when you first start using MCT oil, use a small dose. Taking too much can make you . . . well . . . let's just say head for the bathroom more often (and in more of a hurry) than you prefer.

Can I substitute green smoothies for the broth or the shakes on this diet?

Yes. Feel free to mix and match because you'll still get the phytonutrients and protein you need. In fact, you can swap out anything on this plan—soups for shakes, shakes for green smoothies, green smoothies for soups—you get the picture!

Reminder: You'll find a printable meal plan, a blank meal plan, a shopping list, a list of recommended brands, and lists of "yes" and "no" foods on the Resources page of my website at drkellyann.com/cleansebook.

Chapter 5

After Your Cleanse

Dr. Kellyann's Lifestyle Plan

When you finish your cleanse, you're going to get your freak on . . . and I mean that in a *good* way.

Don't you love that feeling like your feet are barely touching the ground, and you're light as a feather? That's what I'm talking about. You'll have insane energy, you'll feel truly *well* for possibly the first time in years, and you'll keep looking for excuses to peek at your gorgeous skin in the mirror. And if you're like most people who do my cleanse, you're even going to feel a little (ahem) frisky.

So baby, take a moment and completely love on yourself. It just feels so good to conquer a goal, so enjoy it.

But listen . . . we need to talk. It's about that day that's coming: you know, the day *after* your cleanse.

Here's the thing. This "day after" will be the first day of your post-cleanse life—and I want the big wins you get from your cleanse to last a lifetime.

So now, I want to tell you how you can keep the beautiful skin, radiant energy, and healthy body you have now—and how you can keep off any pounds you've lost as well. I call it Dr. Kellyann's Lifestyle Plan, and here's how it works.

First, Get to Your Goal Weight

If weight loss is one of your goals, and you're not at your ideal weight when you finish your cleanse, just switch over to my Bone Broth Diet. This is a simple, gentle diet that you can do for as long as it takes to reach your target. (I have patients who've lost hundreds of pounds on it.)

Alternately, if you only have a few more pounds to lose, and you have a big day coming up—for instance, a wedding or class reunion—you can do my 10-Day Belly Slimdown. It's designed to melt off belly fat *fast*—up to 12 pounds and 5 inches of it.

Once you hit your goal weight, you're ready for the next step.

Say Goodbye to the Foods That Made You Sick and Fat

When you end your cleanse, there's a chance you might be planning to go back to eating a diet centered around low-fat foods and whole grains. That's because you may believe that this diet is good for you.

Not so fast.

The truth is that ever since health "experts" first started promoting this diet decades ago, we've experienced epidemics of obesity and diabetes. Far from getting healthier, we're sicker than we've ever been, and here's why.

First of all, grains—even the so-called healthy ones—turn directly into sugar in your body. (In fact, two slices of whole wheat bread contain as much sugar as a candy bar.) Eat grains at every meal and you'll continually spike your insulin, making you store belly fat. This belly fat, in addition to being unsightly, is a factory that cranks out toxic chemicals that sicken your cells and make you gain even more weight.

The end game here is more inflammation—and inflammation, as I said earlier, is the common underpinning to everything you don't want. It's the fast track to aging, uncontrollable weight gain, and just about every modern-day disease.

What's more, grains contain substances that cause that "leaky gut" I talked about in Chapter 2. In particular, gliadin (a protein in wheat gluten) and wheat germ agglutinin (another protein found in high levels in whole wheat) can increase intestinal permeability and trigger an immune response.[1]

Now, let's talk about what a grain-loaded diet does to your skin. First of all, it promotes acne breakouts. In fact, an article in the *Journal of Drugs in Dermatology* goes so far as to say that carbohydrates are the *main culprit* in acne.[2] But that's just the tip of the iceberg because I've found after decades of clinical experience that a diet high in grains causes flare-ups of psoriasis, eczema, and rosacea as well. (The great news is that cutting out grains frequently clears up my patients' skin like magic.)

Skin problems are a huge issue for a lot of people, and I've witnessed this in my own home. One of my sons suffered from terrible acne, and I saw firsthand how it affected just about every part of his life. After a lot of emotional turmoil, we dialed in to bone broth and omitted dairy and gluten from his diet. It was a beautiful thing to watch the lock-and-key effect—you know, when you finally find the right key that unlocks the door to a solution.

While it's messing with your skin, a diet that's heavy in grains is also messing with your appetite. That's because it makes your brain insensitive to *leptin*, the hormone that tells you when you've had enough to eat. So even when you don't need to eat, you're desperate for food.

Finally, it might surprise you to hear this: grains are a poor source of nutrients, except for the ones that manufacturers add, and you can get the nutrients in grains from better sources. In fact, your body doesn't need grains at all, which is why there's no minimum daily requirement for them. Did you know that? I want to underscore this to you, because people naturally think that grains are part of a healthy diet. But there's NO science that says we need them.

And here's another strike against the high-carb, low-fat diet: while it's overloading you with grains, this diet also shorts you on good fats. Your body desperately needs these nourishing fats to build cell membranes, produce hormones, and keep your brain happy and healthy. Cheat your body of them, and you'll get fat, sluggish, moody, wrinkly, and "brain-foggy."

Also, when you don't get enough fat, you don't get enough of something called *ceramides*. These are fat molecules on the top layer of your skin that make it look soft and moist. So when you're getting wrinkly, it's often the ceramides that you're missing.

In short, a diet that's high in grains and stripped of healthy fats is going to inflame your body, wreck your skin, leave you sad and sick and starving, and pack those pounds right back on you. And all of the benefits you got from your cleanse are going to disappear.

Luckily, the solution is easy: kiss that diet goodbye! Instead, cut down on grains or even eliminate them, and give healthy fats a place in your diet along with clean proteins (including collagen and bone broth), non-starchy veggies, and *small* servings of good carbs in the forms of fruits and starchy veggies.

When you do this, you'll lower your levels of insulin, keep your gut wall strong, beautify your skin, rev up your brain, and banish inflammation. What's more, it'll be easier for you to keep off any pounds you lost during your cleanse.

If you're skeptical about that last promise—and you may be, if you've gained back weight after a previous cleanse or diet—take a look at the latest research, involving one of the biggest studies ever done on long-term weight maintenance.[3]

In this experiment, researchers asked 164 adults to eat one of three maintenance diets—high-carb (60% of total calories), moderate-carb (40% of total calories), or low-carb (20% of total calories)—after they finished a weight-loss diet. The researchers tinkered with the participants' calorie intakes to keep their weights stable and then measured the amount of energy they burned, following them for twenty weeks.

Amazingly, the people on the low-carb plan burned about *250 calories more per day* than those on the high-carb plan. The people in the low-carb group who had the highest insulin secretion at the beginning of the study did even better, burning *up to 478 calories more per day* than the people in the high-carb group.

As an added bonus, the low-carb group had lower levels of a hormone called ghrelin, which stimulates hunger. So they burned more fat and were less hungry!

The biggest takeaway from this study is that "calories in, calories out" is purely a myth. In reality, the *type* of calorie you eat matters—and it's the carbs (especially grain carbs), not the fats or proteins, that pack pounds on you. That's another big reason to kick that high-carb, low-fat diet to the curb.

Say a Big Hello to Dr. Kellyann's Lifestyle Plan!

Now you know which foods will make your post-cleanse glow last for a lifetime. You know that you want to minimize the carbs (especially grains), and maximize the proteins, healthy fats, and veggies that load you with slimming, energizing nutrients.

So . . . are we done? Hold on just a minute, babycakes.

Here's the thing. If you were an annoyingly perfect person, we actually *would* be done now because you'd simply eat the foods that are good for you. However, like me, you're perfectly imperfect. And that means that sometimes—in fact, pretty often—you're going to want to eat foods that are on the "no" list.

Now, you may try to resist your cravings for these foods. But you know what happens when you *can't* have a food? You crave it even more, so eventually you binge on it. Instead of going for a slice of pizza or a scoop of ice cream, you eat the whole pizza or the entire carton of ice cream. And it doesn't take long for those pounds to come back.

Why? Because *you're obsessed with what you can't have.* As the old saying goes, "You get what you focus on." (And boy, do you.) So please . . . don't focus on how you *can't* have pasta, or that's exactly what will end up in your bowl.

You can blame this on a part of your brain called the *reticular activating system.* Here's how it works. Have you ever been at the dinner table and said "Where's the salt?" You get up to look for the salt, and as you're looking, you tell yourself, "I can't find the salt, I can't find the salt, I can't find the salt." What's the result? This is what your mind chooses to focus on. So you can't find the salt.

However, if you get up from the table and think, "I'm going to find the salt," chances are you'll come back with it. Why? Because you're focused on finding it.

Similarly, if you focus your attention on the foods that you consider "taboo," eventually you'll go crazy and stuff your face with them. This is especially true if you're what's called a "restrained" eater—someone who worries a lot about your weight, tends to ignore your hunger cues, and limits taboo foods religiously.[4] (Sound like anyone you know?)

On my lifestyle plan, this isn't going to happen. Cravings aren't going to derail you because you can *have* that ice cream or pizza—or any other naughty food you love—if you're really yearning for it. This is incredibly powerful psychologically.

Now, you may be wondering . . . how can a plan that keeps you healthy and slim forever include the sinful foods you love? It's all about the 80/20 rule. Here's how it works:

- For 80% of your meals, you're going to stick to superfoods that load you with nutrients, keep your blood sugar low, fight inflammation, and rev up your metabolism. And don't worry: these foods are *delicious*. (I'll tell you about them in a minute.) What's more, there's no skimping—you'll fill your plate at every meal.

- For 20% of your meals, you're going to sprinkle on a little "fairy dust" if you want to. As long as you keep your portions reasonable, you can eat any food you desire at these meals. Gelato for lunch? Sure. Your mom's billion-calorie lasagna for dinner? Go for it. As a result, you'll never say "never" to any food you love.

- If you stray from these percentages and wind up feeling blah, looking old, and gaining weight again, you'll be able to erase this damage quickly and easily (more on this later as well, see page 99).

When you eat this way, you're going to put so many credits in your "good food" bank that you can cheat a little without paying any price. I like to say that you're getting 100% of the results for only 80% of the effort.

This is how I live my own life, and I wouldn't have it any other way. It allows me to experience joy. I go out to dinners, I go to cocktail parties, and if I want to indulge in something, I don't put myself through any unneeded torture. Keep this in mind: it's what you do *most* of the time that's going to make a difference. And when you do what's right *most* of the time, you're all good.

Now, let's take a closer look at the two parts of this plan.

Your 80% Meals

For 80% of your meals, you're going to stick to my list of "yes" foods. The good news is that they're fabulous! Here they are:

- Proteins. These include fish, poultry, beef, eggs, organ meats, bone broth, and collagen powder, which will feed your body the amino acids it needs to cleanse, repair, and beautify itself. To make sure you're getting the most nutrients and the least toxins, buy meats that are free from nitrates, nitrites, and sugar, and buy pastured meat and eggs when you can. (When you can't, take the skin off chicken or the fat off beef because that's where most of the toxins collect.)

- Healthy fats. These include clarified butter or ghee, avocados and avocado oil, olives and olive oil, coconut and coconut oil, nuts, and seeds. (You'll find a full list in the 80% template on pages 89 and 90.) Don't skimp, because your body *loves* these fats. And remember those ceramides I talked about that plump up your skin? This is where you'll get them.
- Non-starchy veggies. Load your plate with these—the more, the better. They'll give you the nutrients and fiber you need to stay slender and healthy and battle bloat.
- Small doses of starchy veggies and fruits. These will give you an additional boost of energy any time you need it.

The key here is to be smart about your portion sizes. Simply stick to the 80% template and you can't go wrong.

Your 80% Template

Protein Portions

A serving of meat, fish, or poultry should be about the size and thickness of your palm. A serving of eggs is as many as you can hold in your hand (that's about two or three for women, three or four for men). A serving of egg whites alone is double the serving for whole eggs. Each meal should include a serving of protein.

Non-Starchy Vegetable Portions

A serving of non-starchy vegetables should be at least the size of a softball. These are fabulous for you, so if possible, fill your plate with at least two or three softballs' worth!

Starchy Vegetable Portions

A serving of starchy vegetables (such as sweet potato, jicama, kohlrabi, or winter squash) should be about the size of a baseball for women and the size of a softball for men. Eat these veggies only when you need an extra burst of energy—for instance, on days when you do strenuous workouts.

Fruit Portions

A serving of fruit is half an individual piece (half an apple, half an orange, half a banana) or a tennis ball-size serving of berries, grapes, or tropical fruits (about half a cup). That's a closed fistful if they're diced. Eat no more than two servings of fruit per day and break them up across meals and snacks to distribute your sugar intake.

Fat Portions

A serving of oil or clarified butter is 1 tablespoon.
A serving of nuts, seeds, coconut flakes, or olives is about
  one closed handful.
A serving of nut butter is 1 tablespoon.
A serving of avocado is ¼ to ½ an avocado.
A serving of coconut milk is ⅓ cup.
A serving of chia seeds is 4 teaspoons.
A serving of flaxseed is 2 tablespoons.
A serving of hemp seeds is 2 tablespoons.

To help make your gut glow, I also want you to work *probiotic* and *prebiotic* foods into your meals as often as you can. Probiotics are fermented foods that contain healthy bacteria to reseed your gut; they include kimchi, sauerkraut, and pickles. (Be sure to buy these in the refrigerated case, because the versions on the store shelf are pasteurized, which kills off the bacteria.) Prebiotics are foods that act as fertilizer for your gut bacteria; they include asparagus, onions, jicama, garlic, leeks, Jerusalem artichokes, and unripe bananas.

Oh, and by the way—cocktails are a yes on your 80% days! Just make sure you're drinking smart (see page 106).

Now, you may be wondering why some foods you think of as healthy aren't in the 80% category. Here are the reasons:

- Dairy. The vast majority of my patients discover that dairy products cause bloating, blotchy skin, and other problems. Unless you're sure your body can handle them, you'll want to avoid them.
- Soy. While soy foods are billed as healthy, most of them are "Frankenfoods" loaded with junk. They also contain substances that can mess with your thyroid, putting you at greater risk for autoimmune thyroid disease.[5] By the way, it's not true that people in Asian countries, who are very healthy in general, load up on soy. Instead, they add small amounts of unprocessed soy to their diet as an accent, rather than eating huge amounts of heavily processed soy the way Americans do.
- Seed oils. Oils like corn, canola, and sunflower oil are heavily processed and usually rancid by the time you buy them. In addition, they have high levels of inflammatory omega-6 fatty acids and low levels of anti-inflammatory omega-3 fatty acids. Margarine, which is even more processed and laden with additives, is even worse.

In addition to avoiding these foods, I want you to steer clear of foods with artificial sweeteners or additives. When you shop for your 80% meals, be sure to read labels. If a product's label lists ingredients you can't pronounce, put it back on the shelf. Buy fresh food as often as you can; the fewer bar codes you wind up with in your cart, the better. When you can't go fresh, choose a brand you can trust; see my list of recommended brands on the Resources page of my website at drkellyann.com/cleansebook.

Also, watch out for *hidden* grains. Here's a list of sneaky food additives containing grains; if you see any of these on a product label, it isn't an 80% food.

Sneaky Places Where Grains Hide

Here are some of the ingredients that indicate that a product possibly or definitely contains gluten:

Artificial flavoring
Bleached flour
Caramel color
Dextrin
Hydrolyzed plant protein (HPP)
Hydrolyzed wheat protein
Hydrolyzed wheat starch
Malt
Maltodextrin
Modified food starch
Natural flavoring
Seasonings
Vegetable protein
Vegetable starch
Wheat germ oil
Wheat grass
Wheat protein
Wheat starch

Corn is another grain you'll want to minimize or eliminate—
here are some of its sneaky forms:

Artificial flavoring
Corn alcohol
Corn flour
Corn oil
Corn sweetener
Corn syrup solids
Cornmeal
Cornstarch
Dextrin
Dextrose
Food starch
High-fructose corn syrup
Maizena
Maltodextrin
Modified gum starch
MSG
Natural flavorings
Sorbitol
Vegetable gum
Vegetable protein
Vegetable starch
Xanthan gum
Xylitol

Here's a closer look at the foods to stick to for your 80% meals. I recommend copying this chart and putting it on your fridge so it'll be a
cinch to plan your meals.

Remember: This list is for your maintenance plan. On your cleanse, stick to the meals I outline in Chapter 4. For a printable list of "yes" and "no" foods on Dr. Kellyann's Lifestyle Plan, visit the Resources page on my website at drkellyann.com/cleansebook.

MEATS

Beef	Turkey
Chicken	Wild boar
Lamb	

Note: Buy pastured meat and free-range poultry if you can afford them. If not, remove the skin from the chicken and the fat from the meat (because that's where the toxins collect). Avoid pork unless you can find pastured pork.

FISH AND SEAFOOD

Fresh or canned. Buy wild-caught fish or seafood, if possible, and make sure canned fish or seafood is packed in water or olive oil.

EGGS

Buy free range if possible.

ORGAN MEATS

Look for organic liver.

NITRITE- AND GLUTEN-FREE DELI MEATS, BACON, AND SAUSAGES

Note: Read labels carefully and make sure you're not getting any sugars or artificial additives.

VEGETABLES

Acorn squash
Artichokes
Arugula
Asparagus
Beets
Bell peppers
Bok choy
Broccoli
Broccoli rabe
Brussels sprouts
Butternut squash
Carrots
Cauliflower
Celery
Celery root
Chile peppers
Cilantro
Cucumber
Eggplant
Garlic
Green beans
Green cabbage
Green onions
Greens (beet, collard, mustard, and turnip greens)
Jalapeño peppers
Jicama
Kale

Kohlrabi
Leeks
Lettuce
Mushrooms
Napa cabbage
Onions
Parsnips
Plantains
Radicchio
Radishes
Red cabbage
Rutabaga
Seaweed
Snap peas
Snow peas
Spaghetti squash
Spinach
Sprouts
Summer squash
Sweet potatoes and yams
Swiss chard
Tomatoes (including canned or sun-dried tomatoes)
Turnips
Watercress
White potatoes
Yuca
Zucchini

Notes: Eat starchy vegetables like sweet potatoes and winter squash sparingly. Add them to a meal only if you need extra fuel after a workout or a strenuous day.

Buy organic vegetables if possible.

Corn is a grain and not a vegetable, and it is not on the 80% list.

FRUITS

Apples

Applesauce, unsweetened

Apricots

Bananas

Blackberries

Blueberries

Cantaloupe

Cherries

Dates

Figs

Grapefruit

Grapes

Guava

Honeydew melon

Kiwifruit

Lemons

Limes

Mandarin oranges

Mangoes

Nectarines

Oranges

Papayas

Peaches

Pears

Pineapples

Plums

Pomegranates

Pumpkin

Raspberries

Rhubarb

Strawberries

Tangerines

Ugli fruit

Watermelon

Note: Buy organic if possible; also, emphasize berries and grapefruit, which are lower in sugar than most fruits. Avoid dried fruits and fruit juices.

HEALTHY FATS

Almond butter

Avocado oil

Avocados

Chia seeds

Coconut

Coconut chips

Coconut milk (canned, full-fat)

Coconut oil

Ghee (clarified butter)

Ground flaxseed

Hemp seeds
MCT oil
Nuts
Olive oil

Olives
Tallow
Walnut oil

COLLAGEN AND PROTEIN POWDERS
Collagen protein
Egg protein
Hydrolyzed beef protein
Pea protein (not optimal but okay)

FERMENTED FOODS
Coconut kefir
Kimchi (refrigerated)
Pickles (unpasteurized, refrigerated)
Sauerkraut (refrigerated)

CONDIMENTS
Cocoa powder,
 unsweetened
Coconut aminos
 (to replace soy sauce)
Fish sauce
Herbs
Hot sauce, gluten-free
Mustard, gluten-free
Pepper

Pickles, unsweetened
 and sulfite-free
Salsa
Salt, Celtic or pink
 Himalayan (instead of
 regular table salt)
Spices
Vinegar

Note: While regular table salt contains iodine, it also contains additives you don't want. To get a good supply of iodine, be sure to include sea vegetables (like SeaSnax) and fish in your diet, or take a supplement containing iodine.

FLOURS AND THICKENERS
Almond flour
Arrowroot powder
Coconut flour
Tapioca starch

BEVERAGES

Coffee	Sparkling Water
Collagen coffee	Tea
Detox water	Water
Mineral water	

Now, let's talk about your 20% meals—or, as I call them, your "fairy dust" meals.

What About Beans and Lentils?

You may be wondering if beans and lentils are permitted on the lifestyle plan. Well, it's tricky! This is a gray area because these foods contain high levels of substances called phytates and lectins that some people can't handle well. However, other people do just fine with beans and lentils. So I say, go with what works for you.

Personally, I stick with black beans and lentils—which appear to be the least problematic of the group—adding a little to my diet to increase my intake of resistant starch (see page 95). If you decide to add beans and lentils to your own diet, see how you react to them. If they cause problems for you, make them a 20% food or eliminate them entirely. If not, you can add them in small quantities to your 80% meals.

Your 20% Meals

Several times each week, you can enjoy a favorite food—no matter how wicked—that's not on my list of "yes" foods. All you need to do is stick to reasonable portions and say no to seconds.

Now, a little math shows that 20% of 21 weekly meals works out to roughly four meals. Here's the deal: you can stick with that, or you can limit yourself to fewer fairy-dust meals.

When you're deciding which way to go, ask yourself questions like these:

- How much weight, if any, do you still want to lose? If you're not at your goal weight, you'll reach that goal faster by aiming for 90/10.
- Do you need tweaks to get fit, or do you need a major health overhaul? If you have an autoimmune condition or other serious health problem, it's smart to minimize your fairy-dust meals.

Also, get to know your own body. No two people are alike, and what works for someone else may not work for you. That's why I want you to play detective as you add foods back into your diet. Introduce one food group at a time, waiting several days before introducing another, and explore questions like these:

- Does gluten cause problems for you? When you eat gluten-containing grains, do you experience bloating, brain fog, or other problems? If not, you can introduce small amounts of them back into your diet. Otherwise, give this category of grains a pass even for your 20% meals.
- Do even gluten-free grains affect you in bad ways? If you gain weight easily when you eat grains, or you experience acne, rosacea, or psoriasis, you're better off cutting way back on them or even eliminating them.

- How do you respond to dairy? Odds are, you'll feel and look better if you cut dairy out of your diet. However, some people can handle it just fine. Test cheese and milk separately because some people can tolerate one and not the other.

  One word of warning: some people haven't yet connected the dots between the symptoms they're experiencing and dairy being the cause. So if you're having aches and pains, rashes, headaches, or other symptoms that you haven't quite figured out, you may want to pull dairy even if you think you can tolerate it.

- How do carbs affect your blood sugar? If you have high blood sugar—even if you're not diabetic—you need to watch your carbs very, very carefully. Take your blood sugar measurements on a regular basis and find out how many carbs (and which types of carbs) your body can tolerate. (For more on this, check out my article "How to Measure Your Blood Sugar" on the Resources page of my website at drkellyann.com/cleansebook.)

The clues you uncover through your detective work will help you decide how much fairy dust you can spread, which foods to let back into your life, and which foods to avoid even for your 20% meals.

One more word of advice: try to limit the worst carbs even on your fairy-dust days. Bread and pasta have few nutrients, while junk foods like doughnuts and cake have virtually none. Starchy veggies and fruits are high-quality carbs because they contain lots of nutrients and a good dose of fiber.

So choose starchy veggies over grains and sugar as often as possible, even for your 20% meals. Also, if you decide to add grains back into your diet, stick to organic, non-GMO grains and—when possible—choose grains that are ancient, sprouted, and/or fermented. And opt for rice occasionally, because when you prepare it the right way, it's a good source of resistant starch (see page 95).

What Are Net Carbs?

Different people can eat different amounts of carbs without gaining weight or having blood sugar problems. That's why I recommend getting smart about the number of carbs your own body can handle.

To do that, however, you need to know what *net* carbs are—because that's the number that matters, and here's why.

The carbohydrates in food fall into several categories, which include:

- Fiber
- Starch
- Sugar alcohols
- Sugars

You'll see some, if not all, of these on nutrition labels as well as in nutrient databases and apps such as MyFitnessPal.

The thing to know is that not all categories of carbohydrates affect your blood sugar the same way. For instance, starches and sugars are rapidly absorbed and converted to glucose, which generally causes sharp spikes in your blood sugar and insulin. That's what you want to avoid.

On the other hand, fiber and sugar alcohols are absorbed slowly, if at all. Moreover, they're metabolized differently, if at all. As a result, they don't cause your blood sugar and insulin levels to rise. And that's a good thing!

Thus, the most accurate way to calculate your carb load is to consider only net carbs, or the actual amount of carbs that will affect your blood sugar. Knowing the net carbs of foods will allow you to stay in the right carb range.

Here are a few examples:

Raspberries. Raspberries are an excellent source of antioxidants as well as fiber. A half-cup serving contains approximately 7 grams of carbohydrates. However, 4 grams of this total comes from dietary fiber. So here's the math:

7 grams (total carbs) – 4 grams (dietary fiber) = 3 grams (net carbs)

Spinach. Spinach is packed with vitamins, minerals, and powerful plant nutrients to keep you healthy and slim. I love adding a handful to my collagen shakes. And fortunately, most of the carbs (64%) come from fiber. This means you can get away with eating lots of spinach as well as most other leafy greens. The net carb count for one cup of spinach is as follows:

6.75 grams (total carbs) – 4.32 grams (dietary fiber) = 2.43 grams (net carbs)

Avocado. Avocado is one of my favorite superfoods. It's got it all: healthy fat, vitamins, minerals, phytonutrients, and a good dose of fiber. Plus, it's creamy and delicious! Let's take a look at the numbers for a half-cup serving:

6.4 grams (total carbs) – 5 grams (dietary fiber) = 1.4 grams (net carbs)

Bottom line: to get the whole picture, look for that word *net* when you're adding up your daily carbs.

One More Tip: Check Out Resistant Starches

When you start on the lifestyle plan, there's one type of starch I want you to consider adding to your diet on a regular basis. It's called *resistant starch*, and it's one of the hottest trends in healthy eating. Here's the scoop on what it is and why I make it part of my own meals.

Resistant starch is a type of starch that resists being digested in your small intestine. (That explains its name.) Instead, it's fermented in your large intestine.

There are four types of resistant starch, but only three of them occur naturally. They're type 1 (found in grains, seeds, and legumes), type 2 (found in green bananas, green plantains, and raw potatoes), and type 3 (created in certain starchy foods when you cook and then chill them).

If you eat a typical diet, you're already getting some resistant starch. However, many experts recommend upping your intake. Here are some of the ways in which eating resistant starch can benefit you:

- Because it doesn't break down and get turned into sugar in the small intestine, resistant starch doesn't hike your blood sugar and insulin levels like nonresistant starch does. In fact, research shows that resistant starch improves insulin sensitivity,[6] helping you to lose weight and protecting against diabetes.
- The fermentation process that breaks down resistant starch in your lower intestine creates beneficial molecules including butyrate[7]—that short-chain fatty acid I talked about back in Chapter 2 that lowers your inflammation, helps you burn more fat, and fights cancer.
- Resistant starch acts as "fertilizer" for your gut bugs, fostering a healthy microbiome.[8]
- Because it's high in fiber, resistant starch fills you up so you're less likely to overeat.[9]
- Resistant starch can improve your cholesterol and triglyceride levels.[10]

There are easy ways to increase your intake of resistant starch. For instance, beans and seeds contain a significant level of resistant starch when you cook them in the normal way. A green banana tossed into a shake or a handful of green plantain chips will also give you a good dose of this starch.

However, to get the benefits of resistant starch from foods like potatoes and rice, you need to cook them and then chill them—preferably for at least twenty-four hours. Cooking causes the starch to swell and absorb water, while chilling it causes it to crystallize into a form that resists the digestive process.

The easiest way to use chilled potatoes or rice is in salads—for instance, a classic potato salad made with avocado mayo, or rice tossed with veggies and an olive oil dressing. By the way, beans develop even more resistant starch when they're cooled, so don't just eat them hot—try tossing them into cold salads.

Before you add resistant starch to your diet, however, I do have some cautions:

- If you've been diagnosed with small intestinal bacterial overgrowth (SIBO), resistant starch could worsen the condition. Be sure you heal your gut before adding this starch to your diet.
- Also limit resistant starch if you have irritable bowel syndrome because it could aggravate your symptoms.
- Go slowly. Overloading your gut with resistant starch can cause gas and bloating.
- Get your resistant starch from whole foods, not potato starch. Resistant starch appears to be more beneficial when it's combined with other soluble and insoluble fibers, and there's some evidence that resistant starch eaten in isolated form can actually be bad for you.

And, as always, listen to the wisdom of your own body. Remember that every person—and every body—is unique, and what works for someone else might not work for you. So keeping my cautions in mind, add a little extra resistant starch to your diet and keep close track of your results.

Putting It All Together

To make it easier for you to visualize your 20% meals, here are two samples from different patients of mine. Jane limits herself to three fairy-dust meals each week and likes to save them for the weekends, while Mark eats four fairy-dust meals and spreads them out over the week.

Jane's 80/20 Week

	MON	TUES	WED	THURS	FRI	SAT	SUN
Breakfast	80% Meal	80% Meal	80% Meal	80% Meal	80% Meal	20% Meal: Eggs and hash browns	20% Meal: Pancakes with the kids
Lunch	80% Meal	80% Meal	80% Meal	80% Meal	80% Meal	80% Meal	80% Meal
Dinner	80% Meal	80% Meal	80% Meal	80% Meal	80% Meal	20% Meal: Girls' night out—Shrimp fettucine and one slice of Death by Chocolate cake	80% Meal

Mark's 80/20 Week

	MON	TUES	WED	THURS	FRI	SAT	SUN
Breakfast	80% Meal	80% Meal	80% Meal	20% Meal: Bagel and cream cheese	80% Meal	80% Meal	80% Meal
Lunch	20% Meal: Restaurant meeting with clients— steak and fries	80% Meal	80% Meal	80% Meal	80% Meal	20% Meal: Game-day nachos, wings, and beer	80% Meal
Dinner	80% Meal	80% Meal	20% Meal: Tacos and refried beans with the kids	80% Meal	80% Meal	80% Meal	80% Meal

You might want to create your own calendar to chart your 80% and 20% meals. It's a good way to make sure you're staying on track, especially at first.

Okay, Let's Get Real . . .

Now that you have the lifestyle plan guidelines down pat, let's talk about one more thing—and that's what to do if you sometimes stray way, *way* off the plan.

Here's the deal. I know a lot about life because I've been around for a while. And one thing I know for sure is that every once in a while, you're going to screw up and go on a food binge. And that 80/20 is going to turn into 60/40, 50/50, or maybe even 0/100.

I can't predict when or why it'll happen. Maybe you'll be stressed out over work. Maybe you'll go through a bad breakup. Or maybe it'll be for a happy reason like a family wedding, a vacation, or a holiday. Whatever the cause, sooner or later, you're going to blow it big-time. If you're sad or stressed, you're going to fall face-down into a pint of Cherry Garcia. If you're celebrating, you're going to go overboard on the cheesecake and mojitos. Either way, when you come up for air, you'll be five pounds heavier.

You know what? When this happens, I'm not going to go all preachy on you. That's because if you read Chapter 1, you know I've been there myself. So don't kick yourself if you fall off the 80/20 wagon.

Here's what I've learned from every single winning stallion that I know. They don't let setbacks make them fall. They stand up, brush themselves off, and just go. And this is what I want you to do. Just remember that every day is a new opportunity.

If you fall off the wagon, don't mope, and don't guilt-trip yourself. Instead, simply do one or two bone broth fasts, eating nothing but broth for twenty-four hours each time. (You can drink your broth at any time of the day or night while you're fasting.) This "mini-cleanse" will erase the damage like it never even happened.

Six Tips for Success on Your Maintenance Plan

I've helped thousands of people maintain their wins after cleanses or diets—and in the process, I've identified six of the best strategies for long-term success. Here they are:

1. Beware of portion creep—or, as I like to call it, "portion distortion." While your body needs a good dose of superfoods to stay strong and healthy, it doesn't need an overdose. Resist the urge to stretch your portion sizes, because small cheats add up over time. Be especially careful with nuts because it's far too easy to hoover up a whole can at once.

2. Nip problems in the bud. Don't wait until you're in a downward spiral. The instant you notice that you're not feeling like your best "you" anymore, schedule another cleanse.

3. Keep drinking bone broth and using collagen every day. This habit will give you a healthy gut and beautiful skin for life. Bone broth really is a meal in a mug, and you can drink it straight or add it to soups, stews, or even cocktails. To get your collagen fix, stir it into smoothies or soups, or have a daily cup of my Collagen Coffee.

4. Don't forget those healthy fats. These give you beautiful skin, help to balance your hormones, and keep your metabolism fired up. Don't overdo them, but don't skimp either.

5. Continue to load your diet with healthy greens. That filling fiber keeps cravings at bay, so it's easier to avoid overeating. When you're in a hurry, powdered greens are a great way to add a quick shot of nutrition to shakes and smoothies. For recommended brands of powdered greens, visit the Resources page on my website at drkellyann.com/cleansebook.

6. Take good care of yourself. When you're busy caring for other people, it's easy to neglect your own needs. But *you matter, too.* As I tell my patients, "Love yourself, dammit!" This includes scheduling time every day for exercise, stress-busting activities, and just plain fun.

FAQs

Here are some of the questions I'm asked most often about Dr. Kellyann's Lifestyle Plan.

Q: Why do I need to limit fruits and starchy vegetables?
A: These foods are terrific for you in small doses. However, they're high in carbs that raise your blood sugar and make your body release more insulin—and we want to keep your insulin level low.

As a rule of thumb, I recommend limiting your fruits to one or two small servings each day and eating starchy veggies only when you've worked hard and need an extra dose of energy.

When you do eat fruits, I recommend choosing berries or grapefruit most of the time. Both of these are fairly low in sugar compared to other fruits, and they're packed with fat-burning nutrients. (Just be sure you're not taking any medications that prevent you from eating grapefruit.)

Q: I'm thinking of going vegetarian. Can I replace animal proteins with non-animal proteins on the lifestyle plan?
A: Yes, you can! Here's how to do it:

- Substitute egg, pea, or hemp protein for the beef protein powder in your shakes.
- Enjoy eggs at lots of your meals. In addition, you can stretch the basic diet template to include beans and lentils, edamame, full-fat pastured-milk kefir and yogurt, natto, and tempeh. Make sure any soy products you use are non-GMO.
- Finally, substitute a rich vegetable broth for bone broth. If you're a pescatarian, you can substitute fish broth instead.

Do avoid veggie chicken wings, tofu hot dogs, and the like. Knowledgeable nutritionists call these "Frankenfoods" because they're so far removed from real food that they're virtually unrecognizable. It's like thinking that Apple Jacks have anything to do with an apple.

Q: I'm at my goal weight and don't want to lose any more. How can I eat right and still maintain my weight?
A: Easy! Simply add an extra serving or two of starchy vegetables to your diet each day. This is also a great option if you're very active.

Q: How can I follow the plan when I'm traveling?

A: I live half my life in airports and hotels, so I know it can be a challenge to eat right when you're on the road—but with a little planning, you can do it. Here are my favorite tips:

- Pack some lifesavers like dried bone broth (you can buy it online at my site or others) and collagen powder.
- Take along low-carb snacks like coconut chips and nuts so you won't be tempted by the junk in airport vending machines or food courts.
- If you're eating out with friends or clients, check out restaurant menus online ahead of time. Most restaurants either offer healthy options or are willing to make substitutions for you. (Salads with vinegar-and-olive-oil dressing are a good fallback.) Finally, plan on having a few fairy-dust meals when you're away from home.

Q: I tried adding dairy back into my diet, and you're right—it makes me bloat. But I'm still craving cheese. Do you have any advice?

A: First, realize that cheese is actually addictive. That's because it contains casomorphins, which are morphine-like chemicals that latch on to the same receptors in your brain as narcotics. So you're going to crave cheese like crazy when you first give it up, but over time, your desire for it will fade. Don't hit me when I say that . . . it really *will* fade. In the meantime, here are a couple of fabulous cheese substitutes:

- Check out the new cashew-based cheeses. These even come in a liquid form that's delicious when heated. If they aren't in your stores, you can find them on Amazon. Pair them with Siete grain-free chips and you'll be in heaven.
- Try nutritional yeast. I know it sounds unappealing, but it's actually delicious, with a flavor reminiscent of Parmesan cheese. In addition, it's loaded with B vitamins, so it's super-good for

you. Sprinkle it on veggies (and on popcorn, if that's one of your guilty pleasures).

Q: I'm a grazer by nature. Is it okay for me to add snacks to this plan?
A: If you can avoid snacking, do it. The research shows that snacking is a dead end and that intermittent fasting (see page 109) is a far better way to get results.

Here's why I recommend breaking the grazing habit:

- Snacking keeps your insulin and leptin levels spiking all day long. This can lead to insulin resistance and leptin resistance, adding pounds to your waistline and making you hungry all the time.
- Grazing makes it harder for your body to clear out toxins. When you go for ninety minutes to two hours without eating, the muscles in your small intestine generate a "cleansing wave" that flushes toxins out. When you snack all the time, you deactivate this wave.
- Grazing can promote bloating and constipation. After a large meal, you may feel the need to "go" because cues such as stomach distention tell your GI tract to make room for the food that's about to arrive. When you eat small snacks all day, your gut may not get these cues—and as a result, your plumbing can get sluggish.

I know it can be a little hard at first to stop snacking—but when you substitute bone broth, you'll get the satisfaction of grazing without the downsides.

Q: How will I get enough calcium if I'm not eating dairy foods?
A: It's a myth that dairy foods are your only source of calcium. The table that follows lists other foods that provide you with a good dose of this mineral. If you can't work enough of them into your diet, you can simply take a food-based calcium pill.

FOOD	SERVING SIZE	CALCIUM AMOUNT
Collard Greens, raw	½ cup	32 mg
Kale, raw	½ cup	32 mg
Bok Choy, raw	½ cup	20 mg
Figs, dried	½ cup	96 mg
Turnip Greens, raw	1 cup	80 mg
Spinach, cooked	1 cup	240 mg
Almonds	¼ cup	75 mg
Sesame Seeds	1 Tbsp	22 mg
Sardines (with bones)	1 cup	569 mg
Salmon (with bones)	3 oz.	181 mg
Orange	Medium-sized	60 mg
Acorn Squash (cooked)	1 cup	90 mg
Arugula, raw	1 cup	125 mg
Broccoli, raw	1 cup	112 mg
Okra, raw	1 cup	77 mg
Chicory (curly endive), raw	1 cup	40 mg
Dandelion Greens, raw	1 cup	80 mg
Kale, raw	1 cup	55 mg
Kelp or Kombu	1 cup	60 mg
Mustard Greens	1 cup	40 mg
Cress	1 cup	188 mg
Rhubarb, raw	1 cup	103 mg
Carrots, raw	1 cup	36 mg
Walnuts	¼ cup	28 mg
Hazlenuts	¼ cup	56 mg
Brazil Nuts	¼ cup	53 mg

Sources: ucsfhealth.org/education/calcium_content_of_selected_foods/ and iofbonehealth.org/calcium-calculator

Q: Do you recommend taking supplements?

A: Yes. In particular, I recommend these supplements:

- Vitamin D. One caution, however: before supplementing with this vitamin, get your vitamin D levels checked. Vitamin D is actually a hormone, and you can overdo it and get toxic levels. Most people are critically low, but it's smart to verify first.
- A balanced supplement of omega-3, -6, and -9 fatty acids. These help to keep your skin, your brain, and your hormones happy.
- MCT oil. For more on this, see page 73.
- Probiotics. These will help you keep your gut's ecosystem lush and healthy.
- Ashwagandha. This herb is an *adaptogen* that helps your body adapt to stress. It's great for your thyroid, your blood sugar, and your immune system, and it can help to protect you against depression and anxiety.
- Natural Calm. One dose of this magnesium supplement right before bedtime can help you sleep like a baby.

Also, keep drinking green smoothies every day. Another good diet "hack" is to drink 32 ounces of celery juice on an empty stomach each day because it's an awesome cleanser.

Cheers! A Little Alcohol Can Be Good for You

I'm all about being healthy—but I also believe in living it up a little, and I enjoy the occasional drink. So on Friday nights, you're likely to find me celebrating the end of a long week with a shot of potato vodka.

Luckily, research shows that if you choose to drink, a small amount of alcohol can actually be good for you—and for your waistline. Check out some of the findings that scientists are reporting:

- Researchers collecting data from nearly 20,000 women found that "compared with non-drinkers, initially normal-weight women who consumed a light-to-moderate amount of alcohol experienced smaller weight gain and lower risk of becoming overweight and/or obese during 12.9 years of follow-up."[11]
- In a study involving 108 patients with carotid arteriosclerosis, researchers asked half of the patients to follow a modified Mediterranean diet and to exercise. Within this group, half of the patients drank red wine while the other half avoided alcohol. A second group continued their customary lifestyles, with half drinking red wine and the other half abstaining. The researchers found that a glass of red wine each day had positive effects on cholesterol that were independent of dietary and lifestyle changes.[12]

So go ahead and pour yourself a glass of red wine at dinner or order a cocktail when you're out at a restaurant. However, keep some cautions in mind.

First, avoid overdoing it. Unlike light drinking, heavy drinking can pack pounds on you—and it's terrible for your liver, your skin, and your brain as well.

Remember, too, that your ability to metabolize alcohol will lessen as you age, meaning that you can't drink like you did a decade ago. (Well, technically, you can . . . but you're gonna regret it later on.)

Also, be smart about which booze you choose. Beer is loaded with carbs that will go straight to your belly. It also contains gluten (unless it's specifically labeled as gluten-free), which can cause inflammation. Drinks containing commercial mixers are filled with sugar, which will hike your blood sugar and insulin levels and pack pounds on you.

So avoid beer and sugary mixers. Instead, reach for wine or distilled spirits, and use sin-free mixers like sparkling water or muddled berries. Also, check out "A Healthier Way to Mix: Collagen and Bone Broth Cocktail Recipes," on the Resources page of my website at drkellyann.com/cleansebook. *Salud!*

Chapter 6

More Ways to Keep Your Body Clean, Sexy, and Healthy for Life

This cleanse is a powerful first step in your healing process, but it's just that: the first step toward becoming the best "you" that you can be.

So start with your cleanse, but don't stop there. Instead, keep adding more elements to your self-care plan.

Here are my favorite healing and cleansing strategies. They helped me pick myself up after I hit rock bottom, and they can help you reclaim your health and happiness as well.

Do Mini-Fasts

Earlier, I talked about doing a twenty-four-hour bone broth fast any time you start to feel your cleanse gains slipping away. Now, I want to encourage you to go even further and make intermittent fasting (or, as I like to call it, mini-fasts) a part of your regular lifestyle. This may sound challenging, but it's actually easy—and it's one of the greatest gifts you can give your body.

I know that lots of "experts" tell you to eat three meals a day, every single day. Others even recommend grazing all day long. But in reality, our bodies aren't built for nonstop eating, and we pay a big price for it.

Here's the deal. When it comes to our genes, we're almost identical to our caveperson ancestors. They didn't have a grocery store on every corner, so they went for long periods—often days at a time—without food. As a result, our bodies evolved to use food free time for rest, repair, and rejuvenation. Our overworked cells desperately need this cleansing and healing time, and intermittent fasting provides it to them.

There's a huge body of research showing that intermittent fasting benefits your mind and body. Here are just some of the things that happen when you fast:

- Your levels of human growth hormone (HGH) skyrocket. This "fountain of youth" hormone slims you down, helps you build lean muscle and strong bones, and even boosts your brainpower. During a twenty-four-hour fast, HGH increases an average of 1,300% in women, and nearly 2,000% in men.[1]
- Your levels of insulin plummet and you begin to reverse insulin resistance, lowering your risk for diabetes.
- You reduce inflammation and oxidative stress (damage to your cells caused by destructive molecules).[2]
- You may reduce your risk of Alzheimer's disease. In a 2017 study, researchers showed that intermittent fasting improved cognitive function and prevented deposits of amyloid-B (involved in Alzheimer's) in a mouse model of the disease.[3]
- You increase your levels of brain-derived neurotrophic factor (BDNF), which boosts your brain function and helps to protect you against depression.[4]
- You burn fat more easily and reduce your cravings, allowing you to keep off or take off extra pounds. What's more, you don't need to fast for long periods of time to ramp up your fat burning. One 2017 study involving overweight men and women found

that "time-restricted" eating—in which participants simply ate all of their meals in a shortened time frame (in this case, between 8 a.m. and 2 p.m. each day)—increased fat burning during part of the night and reduced hunger swings during the day.[5] And a 2018 study found that people who simply ate their breakfast ninety minutes later and their dinner ninety minutes earlier reduced their body fat by nearly 2% over the course of ten weeks.[6] (For more on this, see my article on "Fat Burning vs. Fat Storing Hormones" on the Resources page of my website at drkellyann.com/cleansebook.)

- You may even live longer! One classic study showed that rats fasting every other day lived 83% longer than non-fasting rats.[7] A newer study in 2018 found that simply going food-free for an increased number of hours each day, without reducing calorie consumption, increased the life expectancy of mice.[8]

There are lots of different ways to do mini-fasts. Here are my two favorites:

- Once or twice each week, do a twenty-four-hour bone broth mini-fast. During this time, have nothing but bone broth, water, tea, or coffee.
- Follow a time-restricted eating plan. In this approach, you eat all of your daily meals within a certain time window, preferably limiting this window to a maximum of nine hours. For instance, if you eat breakfast at 8 a.m., you'll stop eating by 5 p.m.

I know that fasting can sound a little scary if you haven't tried it. However, both bone broth mini-fasts and time-restricted eating are easy and painless because you can always satisfy your cravings with a mug of broth. As a result, you get all of the benefits without the suffering.

If you want to learn more, check out the article "My Top Ten Tips for Intermittent Fasting" on the Resources page of my website at drkellyann.com/cleansebook.

Drink Clean Water

Filtering your water is one of the easiest steps you can take to keep your body healthy, and it's also one of the most important ones. That's because the water that comes from your tap can be contaminated with everything from pesticides to fire retardants to bleach.

Also, while I don't want to gross you out here, lots of medications wind up in the sewer system and then in your drinking water. Among the drugs that currently contaminate tap water in major U.S. cities are asthma medications, sex hormones, antibiotics, anti-convulsant drugs, pain medications, and tranquilizers.[9]

Luckily, it's easy to clean up your water. A full-house water filtration system is the most effective method—but if you can't afford that, put filters on your faucets and in your bath. If you're really pinching pennies, at least use a water filtration pitcher for your drinking water.

Also, avoid bottled water whenever you can. When the Environmental Working Group analyzed ten major brands of bottled water, they found contaminants in every single one, ranging from radioactive pollutants to arsenic to harmful bacteria.[10] What's more, hormone-altering chemicals can leach from the plastic bottles into the water.

The simplest solution is to invest a few dollars in a stainless-steel water bottle and fill it with filtered water. It'll guarantee that your water is squeaky-clean, and as a bonus, it will save you lots of money over time.

Go Organic (Without Breaking the Bank)

While I love fruits and veggies, I don't love getting a big dose of pesticides and herbicides from non-organic produce. The average sample of non-organic strawberries tested by the Environmental Working Group, for instance, tested positive for more than seven separate pesticides, and some samples tested positive for more than twenty![11] (How creepy is that?)

Pesticides and herbicides may mess with your hormones, your nervous system, and your immune system, and even increase your risk for cancer.[12] One recent study found that people eating the most organic food were 25% less likely to develop cancer than people eating little or no organic food—and even participants eating an otherwise not-so-healthy diet lowered their cancer risk by going organic.[13]

There's an obvious way to keep pesticides and herbicides out of your body: swap out regular produce for organic. However, I know that if you're on a tight budget, *organic* can translate into *too expensive*. Luckily, I have good news for you. You don't need to shop in the organic section for all of your produce. Instead, go organic when it matters most.

To do this, simply use the Environmental Working Group's Dirty Dozen and Clean 15 lists as a guide. Here's how their latest lists stack up.

The Dirty Dozen
These are heavily contaminated, so buy organic varieties if at all possible:

1. Strawberries
2. Spinach
3. Kale
4. Nectarines
5. Apples

6. Grapes
7. Peaches
8. Cherries
9. Pears
10. Tomatoes
11. Celery
12. Potatoes

The Clean 15

These are the least contaminated types of produce, so you can feel pretty confident buying non-organic versions:

1. Avocados
2. Sweet corn
3. Pineapples
4. Frozen sweet peas
5. Onions
6. Papayas
7. Eggplants
8. Asparagus
9. Kiwis
10. Cabbages
11. Cauliflower
12. Cantaloupes
13. Broccoli
14. Mushrooms
15. Honeydew melons

In addition to going organic when you buy the Dirty Dozen fruits and veggies, choose organic herbs when they're available. Even better, consider growing your own herbs. When your rosemary and basil come from your own garden or windowsill, you know exactly what's in them (and what isn't).

Eat Local!

Eating locally grown fruits and veggies is a big trend right now, and I'm very happy about that. That's because being a *locavore* is a healthy practice.

One reason is that fruits and veggies don't have to travel very far. This matters a lot when it comes to nutritional value because the nutrient content of produce starts to diminish immediately after harvesting and continues to drop over time. The farther your tomato or apple needs to travel, the less nutritious it is.

In addition, imported foods often come from countries where the use of pesticides isn't tightly regulated. In some cases, pesticides that are banned in the United States are used. Higher levels of heavy metals may be present in the soil in these countries, and produce may be sprayed with harmful chemicals solely to preserve them while they're in transit.

So buy local produce whenever you can. In particular, shop at farmers' markets where you can actually get to know the people who grow your food.

Buy Pastured Meat and Eggs When You Can

Cows and chickens want to graze and peck happily in green fields, not spend their lives in crowded factory farms getting overdosed on antibiotics. And what's good for them is good for us as well, because pastured meat, poultry, and eggs have far more nutrients than factory-farmed proteins. For instance:

- Pastured beef is richer than factory-farmed beef in conjugated linoleic acid, a powerful cancer fighter and lean muscle builder.[14]
- Pastured eggs contain more skin-smoothing, brain-protecting omega-3 fatty acids than eggs from factory farms. In addition,

they're higher in vitamin E. A study comparing caged hens to free-range hens found that the amount of vitamin E in the yolks of eggs from free-range hens was about twice as high as the amount in the yolks of eggs from caged hens.[15]

- Pastured poultry has more vitamin E than factory-farmed poultry, as well as a far better ratio of anti-inflammatory omega-3 fatty acids to inflammatory omega-6 fatty acids.

Moreover, while pastured animals receive virtually no antibiotics, their meat is far less likely than factory-farmed meat to contain dangerous bacteria. Here's what an investigation by *Consumer Reports* found:[16]

One of the most significant findings of our research is that beef from conventionally raised cows was more likely to have bacteria overall, as well as bacteria that are resistant to antibiotics, than beef from sustainably raised cows [cows raised without antibiotics and preferably grass-fed and/or organic]. We found a type of antibiotic-resistant S. aureus bacteria called MRSA (methicillin-resistant staphylococcus aureus), which kills about 11,000 people in the U.S. every year, on three conventional samples (and none on sustainable samples). And 18% of conventional beef samples were contaminated with superbugs—the dangerous bacteria that are resistant to three or more classes of antibiotics—compared with just 9% of beef from samples that were sustainably produced. We know that sustainable methods are better for the environment and more humane to animals. But our tests also show that these methods can produce ground beef that poses fewer public health risks.

I know that pastured meat, poultry, and eggs are a little pricier than their factory-farmed counterparts—but your health is worth it, isn't it? Also, some cuts of pastured meat—for instance, ground beef and chicken legs—are fairly cheap, and pastured eggs only cost a few dollars more per carton. You can save even more money by buying directly from farmers and ranchers in your area; to locate them, go to eatwild.com.

A Word About Fish

There's been a lot of worry lately about the mercury in wild-caught fish. However, fish—especially oily fish—is incredibly good for you. Oily fish is a great source of omega-3 fatty acids, and it's rich in some nutrients (for instance, iodine and selenium) that can be hard to get from other foods.

My advice: steer clear of the types of fish that are highest in mercury, especially if you're pregnant. These include king mackerel, marlin, orange roughy, shark, swordfish, tilefish, and bigeye tuna. Instead, go for clams, cod, crab, flounder, haddock, lobster, oysters, perch, plaice, pollock, salmon, sardines, scallops, shad, shrimp, sole, squid, tilapia, freshwater trout, and canned light tuna.

Also, choose wild-caught fish if you can. It's higher in nutrients and lower in fat than farm-raised fish, and it's not contaminated with antibiotics.

Toss Out "Dirty" Makeup, Skin-Care Products, and Household Cleaners

Remember this simple rule: what gets *on* your skin goes *through* your skin. This means that chemicals in any product that touches your skin, from your lip gloss to your fabric softener, can enter your bloodstream. And you wouldn't believe some of the dangerous stuff that manufacturers put in these products.

Let's start with makeup. Now, I know I'm treading on sacred ground here. Believe me, I love my lipstick and moisturizer as much as you love yours. And like you, I have favorite brands that I've adored for years and years and years.

These days, however, I'm crossing many of my old faves off my list. That's because I now know the dirty truth about what's in them.

Lots of cosmetics and skin-care products, for instance, contain Teflon. Yes, I'm talking about the same toxic coating that's used for nonstick pans and that's linked to cancer and thyroid disease. Recently, it showed up in sixty-six types of makeup and skin-care products tested by the Environmental Working Group.

Then there are phthalates and parabens, two types of hormone disruptors that can raise your risk of breast cancer and reproductive problems. They're common in cosmetics, lotions, body washes, and nail polish. And speaking of nail polish, many brands contain formaldehyde, a carcinogen, and toluene, a toxin that can affect unborn children.

There's a good chance that your deodorant is brimming with toxins, too. It may contain aluminum, parabens, and propylene glycol (an ingredient in antifreeze). It may also contain two chemicals called TEA and DEA, which have been banned in Europe because they're known carcinogens.

And don't get me started on detergents, fabric softeners, and those scents you spray to cover up the smell of your dog. If you want to know what's in them, Google it and be prepared to be horrified.

I'm not trying to frighten you here. Instead, I want to inspire you to take action by "greening" your makeup, skin-care products, and household cleaners. Here are some good ways to do this:

- Look for fragrance-free products. Many of the most toxic ingredients in cosmetics, skin creams, and household cleaners are fragrances.

- Check out the Environmental Working Group's Skin Deep database to find clean brands of makeup and consult their Guide to Healthy Cleaning to get the inside story on good and bad cleaning products.

- Switch to cleaner products without emptying your wallet by following my swap-a-week plan. Every week or so, when you run out of one "dirty" product, replace it with a cleaner version. When you buy healthier products one at a time, it'll be easy on your budget.

- Go natural. Freshen your air with essential oils, clean surfaces with vinegar and lemon oil, and freshen rugs and carpets with baking soda.

Do High Intensity Interval Training (HIIT) and Lift Weights

You already know that exercise is good for you—but did you know that it's one of the world's most effective anti-aging drugs? It's a fact: simply working out can make you younger on the cellular level.

If that sounds too good to be true, check out the results of a recent study.[17] In it, researchers analyzed the telomeres of nearly 6,000 people. Telomeres are the caps on the ends of your chromosomes (I talked about them back in Chapter 2), and as you age, they get shorter and shorter, putting you at greater risk for dying or developing age-related diseases.

In this study, after adjusting for a variety of factors such as smoking, obesity, and alcohol use, the researchers found that people who exercised the most had much longer telomeres than sedentary people. In fact, the difference amounted to about nine years of cellular aging!

Larry Tucker, one of the scientists involved in the study, commented, "We all know people who seem younger than their actual age.

We know exercise can help with that, and now we know that part of that may be because of its effect on our telomeres."

Other researchers are uncovering still more age-defying effects of working out. In one study, scientists compared 125 amateur cyclists to people who didn't do regular exercise. While the cyclists were all fifty-five or older, they had the muscle mass and cholesterol levels of people decades younger—and their immune systems looked like those of young people, too. In addition, the male cyclists had testosterone levels similar to younger men.[18]

All exercise is good for you, but some forms are extra-good. Two of the best are high-intensity interval training (HIIT) and resistance training with weights. Here's why I'm hoping you'll make them part of your workout routine.

HIIT

In HIIT workouts, you alternate between intervals of high-intensity and low-intensity exercise. For instance, you may sprint as hard as you can on your bike for twenty seconds and then pedal slowly for one minute, repeating these intervals multiple times.

HIIT ramps up your levels of human growth hormone, the anti-aging hormone I talked about a little earlier, by up to 450%.[19] In addition, it causes your cells to make more proteins for your mitochondria (the "power plants" of your cells), slowing the aging process. In one study, researchers compared young and old exercisers to sedentary peers. They found that younger participants doing HIIT had a 49% increase in mitochondrial capacity, while older participants had an astonishing 69% increase.[20]

What's more, HIIT burns fat like crazy. Researchers looking at the effects of HIIT involving bicycle sprints found that it causes the body to release high levels of a group of hormones called catecholamines, which drive the release of abdominal fat.[21]

Resistance Training

In resistance training, you use weights, stretch bands, or the weight of your own body to work your muscles against resistance. Resistance training actually creates microscopic tears in your muscles, and when your body repairs these tears, your muscles become stronger.

Research shows that resistance training is one of the best strategies you can use to fight aging. In one study, for instance, researchers took muscle biopsies from young and old participants, had them do resistance training for twenty-six weeks, and then took new muscle biopsies. Amazingly, a whole host of genes associated with aging had reversed their expression in both young and old participants—meaning that these people didn't just slow but actually began to reverse the aging process![22] I don't know about you, but I'm *totally* on board with something that will turn back the clock like that.

Want Even More Gains from Your Workouts?

Here's a trick that serious athletes use all the time to stay slim and sculpted: exercise while you're fasting, not soon after a meal.

About six hours after a meal, your body enters a fasting state. When this happens, it burns off its stored sugar and then starts breaking down fat and converting it into ketone bodies for fuel. In other words, you start burning fat instead of sugar for energy.

When you exercise in this fasted state, it *blasts* the fat off you. In fact, research shows that if you work out before eating breakfast rather than afterward, you can burn nearly 20% more fat.[23]

Get Enough Sleep

Yeah, I know. When your to-do list is ten miles long, getting enough sleep seems like the impossible dream. (No pun intended.) But if you can tack even an extra half-hour onto your nightly slumber, it will do wonders for you.

Here are just some of the reasons not to short yourself on sleep:

- A study involving more than 1,600 adults found that people who slept six hours a night had more belly fat than those who slept for nine hours. In addition, they weighed more and had lower levels of HDL cholesterol (the heart-healthy "good cholesterol").[24]
- Another study revealed that restricting the sleep of healthy young people for four nights decreased the sensitivity of their fat cells to insulin by 30%, leading to levels typically seen in obese or diabetic people. One of the researchers commented, "This is the equivalent of metabolically aging someone ten to twenty years just from four nights of partial sleep restriction. Fat cells need sleep, and when they don't get enough sleep, they become metabolically groggy."[25]
- Other research indicates that sleep deprivation is associated with an increased risk for colorectal cancer, dementia, depression, anxiety, and heart disease.[26]

So try turning off the TV or skipping a few chores so you can turn in as early as possible. Also, try these tips for improving your sleep:

- Stick as closely as you can to a consistent bedtime schedule.
- Turn off your devices at least an hour before bedtime, or use blue-light-blocking glasses (see the next section) when you look at them.
- Keep your room temperature comfortably cool.

- Use a fan or a white noise machine to mask annoying sounds, and use blackout curtains to keep your room as dark as possible.
- In the evening, well before your bedtime, journal about your problems and possible solutions to them. Hashing things out before you turn in can help you avoid those worries that keep you awake at 2 a.m.

Also, if you think you might have sleep apnea, get tested. Untreated sleep apnea is a major risk factor for obesity, diabetes, heart disease, and depression.

Wear Blue Light Glasses at Night or When Using Your Devices

Not all light is alike—and blue light, which helps to regulate your circadian rhythm during the daytime when you're outside, can mess with your body's internal clocks big-time if you're staring at a computer screen all day or glued to your phone at night. That's because the blue light from these devices suppresses your body's output of melatonin, a hormone that's crucial to regulating your day-night cycle.

In one study, researchers compared the effects of six-and-a-half hours of exposure to blue light to the same amount of exposure to green light. The blue light suppressed melatonin around twice as long as the green light and shifted circadian rhythms by twice as much (three hours compared to one-and-a-half hours).[27]

Luckily, there's a simple fix: just wear blue-blocking glasses when you're using your computer or other devices, especially at night. And if you're a fashionista, don't worry; while the early versions of blue-blocking glasses were ugly as sin, the new ones are much more stylish.

Practice Mindful Meditation

I'm a huge believer in meditation, and I can tell you that slacking off on it was one of the big mistakes that led to my airplane crisis. I've learned my lesson, and these days, I make time to meditate no matter how busy I am. That's because I appreciate the power of the mind-body connection—and I know that to keep my body healthy, I need to get my mind in the game.

If you aren't doing mindful meditation yet, I hope you'll start scheduling fifteen to thirty minutes at least two or three times a week to start doing it. Here are just some of the things that meditating does for you:

- It decreases your levels of the stress hormone cortisol.[28]
- It dampens the activity of genes associated with inflammation.[29]
- It's associated with beneficial changes in brain regions involved in learning, memory, and emotion regulation.[30]
- It reduces pain.[31]
- When incorporated into a program including yoga and other mindfulness-promoting activities, it is as effective as antidepressant medication in preventing a recurrence of depression.[32]

What's more, mindful meditation is simple. Here's how you do it:

- Find a quiet place where you won't be interrupted.
- Get into a comfortable position in a chair or on the floor. Rest your hands on your thighs and close your eyes.
- Notice how you feel. Are you cool or warm? Comfortable or tense? Energetic or tired? Also, notice how your clothes feel against your skin.
- Tune in to your surroundings. What do you hear? What do you smell?
- Let your mind wander where it will. Initially, it will probably go

off in all directions, zooming in on all of your worries. Don't try to stop it. Instead, just examine each thought without judging it, and then gently let it go.

- Focus on your breathing. Take deep breaths in, as if your abdomen is a balloon you're filling with air. Then slowly let each breath out. When your mind wanders, acknowledge your thoughts and release them, and then re-focus your attention on your breathing.
- Try saying a soothing word or sound as you breathe out.

While it's not difficult, mindful meditation is a skill, and it gets easier with practice. At first, you may have trouble simply *being* when you're used to always *doing*. Be patient and you'll get the hang of it.

Practice Deep Breathing

When you're stressed, you tend to breathe shallowly. This can make you anxious, which makes you breathe more shallowly, starting a vicious cycle. Shallow breathing also prevents you from getting stale air out of your lungs.

In contrast, deep breathing—also called *abdominal breathing* or *primal breathing*—triggers a relaxation response in your body. This response actually *alters your gene expression* in ways that reduce inflammation, improve your metabolism, and lower your insulin levels. In addition, deep breathing clears your mind, lowers your blood pressure, helps clean toxins out of your system, and strengthens your immune system.

You can practice deep breathing anytime, anywhere—I like to do it to relax myself before I do an interview or go on TV—and it's easy. Here's how to do it:

- Get into a comfortable position.
- Inhale deeply through your nose for the count of five. Be sure to

"belly breathe," expanding your belly as much as possible. It may help to visualize your belly inflating like a balloon.

- Pause for two counts and then exhale through your mouth. Rather than forcing the air out, release it slowly to the count of five, pulling your belly button back toward your spine. Pause for two seconds before breathing in again.
- If you like, say a soothing word or syllable each time you breathe out.
- Repeat your deep breaths about ten times, and you'll feel the relaxation response kicking in.

Practice deep breathing at least a few times each day to make it a habit. Also, use it to calm yourself before stressful events like a job interview.

Take Saunas

Every week during my recovery I scheduled a sauna, and these days I make time for one whenever I have the chance. That's because saunas aren't just relaxing—they're also strong medicine, and here's why.

First, if you're pegging the stress meter, taking a sauna will lower your levels of the stress hormone cortisol.[33] In addition to easing your anxiety, this will help you lose the "cortisol tire" that forms on your belly when you're chronically stressed.

Moreover, saunas can help you sweat out toxins. While your liver and kidneys are the primary organs responsible for detoxifying your body, research shows that perspiration can also help to remove arsenic, cadmium, lead, and mercury from the body.[34] In addition, sweating can help you rid your body of the toxic plastic additive BPA.[35]

Saunas also can lower your blood pressure,[36] and long-term sauna use can reduce your levels of C-reactive protein—a marker for inflammation.[37] If you have type 2 diabetes or prediabetes, you have still another good reason to take regular saunas: they can lower your blood glucose levels.[38] Finally, taking saunas is linked to a reduced risk of dementia and Alzheimer's disease.[39]

In my case, I chose to use an *infrared* sauna. This type of sauna, which uses light to heat your body directly without heating the air around you, is a great option if you find it hard to tolerate the heat of a steam sauna. As a bonus, infrared saunas also rejuvenate your skin, reducing wrinkles and sun damage.[40]

So do yourself a favor and get in the sauna habit. Nearly every gym has a sauna, and it alone is worth the price of your membership.

Do "Dry Brushing"

Dry brushing is a very simple way to unclog your pores, improve your circulation, reduce cellulite, and stimulate your lymph system to remove toxins. It also gives you an all-over massage, relaxing and destressing you, and it makes your skin glow by removing dead cells.

Here's how to do it:

Use a bristle brush that's designed for dry brushing. (Better yet, buy a kit that contains several brushes, including a special brush for your face.) Your brush should have a long handle so you can reach all areas of your body.

Standing naked in the tub, brush your body, starting with the soles of your feet and moving upward to your heart. Then brush your hands, arms, face, neck, and back, always brushing toward your heart. Be sure to cover every part of your body, being very gentle when you brush areas that are sensitive.

When you're done brushing, take a warm shower. Then pat yourself dry and apply a good skin cream or oil.

Commune with Nature

Do you spend all day in a car, in an office, or in the house? If so, find some time to visit a park, take a hike, or do some gardening. Your mind and body are genetically engineered to crave a regular fix of nature, and they'll love you for it. Here's some of the research on the benefits of letting the outdoors back into your life:

- Scientists in Japan collected data on 280 people who walked either through a city or through a forest. They found that the "forest bathers," as they called them, lowered their cortisol levels, their pulse rate, and their blood pressure.[41]
- In another study, researchers found that "forest bathing" enhanced the activity of natural killer cells, which are key components of the immune system, and elevated the expression of anti-cancer proteins.[42]
- A review of thirty-five different studies found evidence that exposure to "blue spaces"—for instance, lakes, rivers, or the ocean—benefits mental health and well-being.[43]

Being outdoors in nature reduces your stress and gives you a dose of vitamin D, but that's not all. When you're around plants, you're breathing *phytoncides*—airborne chemicals that the plants emit to protect them from insects and germs—and these appear to benefit people as well.[44]

If you don't have a chance to get a regular dose of nature, consider buying a grounding mat you can use indoors. Grounding can give you some of the same benefits as being outdoors; for instance, a recent controlled study found that grounding can improve mood, reduce fatigue, and relieve pain.[45]

When you're seeking a dose of nature, invite animals as well as plants into your life. Think about adopting a pet or volunteering at a shelter—or, if you already have a pet, spend more time playing with it. Being around animals helps to lower your blood pressure, cholesterol, and triglycerides, as well as making you less lonely.[46]

Make Something with Your Hands

These days, we're all about swiping screens or pushing buttons on a remote. But here's a suggestion for making your life happier: put down your devices for at least an hour each day and create something with your hands. Try a new recipe, paint a picture, plant some flowers, or learn a new piece on the piano. In addition to being fun, this physical work can give you a greater sense of resilience and even help to protect you from depression.

Neuroscientist Kelly Lambert says that our brains derive a deep sense of satisfaction and pleasure when we do physical work that produces something tangible, visible, and meaningful. "After all," she says, "nature needed a way to keep the earliest humans from becoming 'cave potatoes.'" She believes that physical labor is so rewarding for the brain that a lack of it contributes to depression, reduced confidence, and a lack of resilience.

To test her theory, Lambert and her team of researchers divided rats into two groups. One group of rats, called the "working rats," had to search hard to locate Fruit Loops hidden in mounds of cage bedding. Another group, dubbed the "trust fund rats," got their Fruit Loops even if they did nothing.

Later, the researchers tested how well the rats performed on a test that involved removing a Fruit Loop from a plastic cat toy ball. The task, Lambert says, was designed to test the rats' boldness and persistence—two qualities strongly linked to success when life gets challenging.

The researchers found that the worker rats spent about 60% more time trying to get the Fruit Loops than the trust fund rats, and made 30% more attempts to get the Fruit Loops. "In their own way," Lambert says, "the worker rats were telling us that their prior training sessions had made them more confident that they could overcome the challenge and retrieve the reward."

She concludes that hands-on work that allows us to see the connection between effort and consequence "is a kind of mental vitamin that helps build resilience and provides a buffer against depression."[47] And that's something that texting or binge-watching Netflix can't do for you.

Get a Massage

Massage is truly coming into its own these days, with more and more people realizing that it can heal the mind and body. While it's a potent stress-buster, that's just one of the benefits of getting a massage. Here are others:

It reduces your blood pressure.[48]

It enhances your mental well-being.[49]

It can improve your quality of sleep. (In fact, one recent study found that it's more effective than the sleep-promoting drug estazolam.)[50]

It can help to reduce symptoms of fibromyalgia.[51]

It can reduce pain and moodiness resulting from premenstrual syndrome.[52]

In addition, research shows that couples massage is a great way for stressed partners to improve their health and relationship. Massage can also help children sleep better, which can translate into better sleep for you as well. So make massage a family affair, and everyone will be happier for it.

Journal

Writing your thoughts down is one of the best ways to clarify your thinking, solve stubborn problems, and relieve stress—and remarkably, there's even evidence that it can make you healthier.

According to psychologist James Pennebaker, an expert on the effects of expressive writing (that is, journaling about feelings and experiences), "The most striking research on expressive writing has been done with markers of physical health and biological changes. We know from multiple studies that there are enhancements in immune function, drops in blood pressure, improvements in sleep, and drops in other markers of stress. People go to the doctor less in the months after [starting] expressive writing. Other studies find faster wound healing, greater mobility among people with arthritis, and the list goes on."[53]

You can either use a pen and paper to journal or do it on your computer. To make your journaling stress-free, relax and let the words flow without fretting over punctuation and spelling. Also, write only for as long as you want—even if it's just for five or ten minutes a few times a week.

Finally, consider starting a "gratitude journal." When you take time to list the people and things for which you're grateful, it can help you focus on the positive rather than on the negative.

Use Essential Oils

Essential oils are highly concentrated, non-water-soluble phytochemicals distilled from different parts of plants. Traditional cultures have used them as medicines for centuries, and they're trendy today because we're rediscovering their healing properties.

I love essential oils, and I use them for everything from promoting sleep (by splashing a little lavender oil in my bath) to fighting infections (by adding a few drops of oregano oil to my bone broth). Used correctly, essential oils can also help you balance your hormones, improve your immune system, and even reduce psoriasis outbreaks.

If you decide to start using essential oils, I strongly recommend doing some research first. A good place to start is with *The Healing Power of Essential Oils* by my friend and colleague Dr. Eric Zielinski, one of the leading experts in the field.

Try Flotation Therapy

If you're out-of-your-mind stressed and you have a little extra money to spare, take an afternoon off and do flotation therapy. In this therapy, you lie in a light- and sound-proof cocoon filled with water that's loaded with enough Epsom salts to make you float. The combination of sensory deprivation, floating, and the magnesium from the Epsom salts eases your stress like magic, and it's great for relieving aches and pains as well.

Don't have enough money to try flotation therapy? Then pour two cups of Epsom salts into a warm bath, along with some lavender oil. You'll get a similar effect for pennies.

Experiment with Acupuncture

Acupuncture is a fabulous stress reliever. It lowers your body temperature, slows your heart beat and respiration, and melts away muscle tension.

In addition, research shows that acupuncture can help fight depression. In one study, for instance, researchers looked at the effects of acupuncture or counseling on 755 people with moderate or severe depression. The researchers found that both approaches were beneficial, lowering scores on a scale measuring depressive symptoms from an average of 16 out of 27 at the start of the study to 9 for acupuncture and 11 for counseling. One in three patients was no longer depressed after three months of acupuncture or counseling, compared to one in five who received neither treatment.[54]

And here's a surprising finding: acupuncture can improve your insulin sensitivity! As I explained in Chapter 2, this is a huge key to staying slim and healthy. In one study involving overweight diabetics, researchers tested the effects of the diabetes drug metformin alone and in combination with acupuncture. They found that the metformin-acupuncture combo was more effective than the drug alone, "proving that acupuncture is an insulin sensitizer."[55]

If you're feeling a little nervous about getting needles stuck in you, acupressure is a noninvasive alternative that's been shown to reduce pain[56] as well as ease depression and sleep problems.[57]

Play!

When we're kids, we spend hours playing Clue, Hula-Hooping, riding bikes, and running races. Then we grow up and get serious, and we put the fun and games behind us. Turns out, that's a mistake.

Just like children, we need to have play in our lives. It relaxes us, helps us shrug off stress, gives us a chance to bond with our friends and family, and even keeps our brains sharp. In short, adults need recess, too.

So let your hair down. Play badminton with your kids, color a picture in an adult coloring book, or challenge your partner to a game of Twister. You're never too old to have fun.

Learn How to Say "NEXT"

Let's face it: life is painful. It doesn't matter if you're rich, poor, young, old, whatever. Life is going to kick you in the teeth sometimes.

The question is: What do you do when it happens?

Here's my best advice: if someone or something hurts you, *dismantle the pain quickly.* This is the best skill I have ever learned. Let yourself understand your pain, face it, process it, get angry—then replace it quickly.

Here's how to do it. First, literally say in your mind . . . *NEXT.* Picture the word.

Next, replace the pain with something that brings you joy. In my case, I picture all of those times when my boys were babies and would crawl all over me like little puppies. I would strap them on me when I went to work, and it is one of the best memories I have.

Find something similar that fills you with joy. This will flood your body with "feel good hormones" and change your state.

Finally, allow yourself to think about your pain once a day at the same time of day—and *only once a day*—for ten minutes. Then you are done.

If you find that someone has done something hurtful to you, NEXT . . . If you find someone doesn't appreciate something about you, NEXT . . . If you bomb a meeting, a job opportunity, NEXT . . . If someone breaks your heart (and this is the toughest), pull out the biggest NEXT you have.

This skill is incredibly important if you want to be happy and healthy. Every structure and function of the body depends on your brain and nervous system. You can't have a good life without having mental peace. And one of the biggest keys to that peace is to let go of the hurts so you can make room for the joys.

Last but (Definitely) Not Least: Respect Yourself

When things start to fall apart, it's often because you're making the mistake of valuing everyone else but not yourself. You're worrying about the people around you—your partner, your kids, your boss—and at the same time you're neglecting your own needs. That's exactly what I was doing before my collapse, and I know just where it leads.

When you constantly put yourself last, it sets off a cascade of negatives. You don't eat right. You short yourself on sleep. You work too hard and play too little. You're stressed all the time, and happy virtually none of the time.

If this sounds like your life right now, here's what I want you to do: *honor* yourself. Realize that you are as important as everyone else in your life and act accordingly.

Instead of saying "yes" to every obligation, say "no" to time-sucking responsibilities that aren't necessary. While you're at it, also shoo negative people out of your life whenever you can. Ask for support from your friends and family rather than always being the rock they depend on. And no matter how busy you are, make your own health and happiness a top priority.

Some of the strategies I've talked about here—drinking clean water, eating clean food, working out, getting the toxins out of your home, and respecting yourself—are absolutely essential if you truly want to be well. When it comes to the rest of them, I'm a believer in "personal play," so pick and choose what works best for you.

The most important thing is to care for yourself—whether you're choosing healthy foods, taking time for a massage, taking a walk in the park, or saying "no" to unnecessary obligations. *You matter,* so make this a key rule for your lifestyle plan: stop putting everyone else first, and start being your own BFF!

PART 3

Recipes for Your Cleanse and Beyond

Chapter 7

Glorious Green Smoothies

One of the hardest-working appliances in my kitchen is my blender. That's because at least once a day, I treat myself to a cool, refreshing, cell-cleansing green smoothie.

On this cleanse, you'll go one better and enjoy *two* green drinks each day. These nutrition bombs are going to saturate your cells with phytonutrients that will make them stand up and dance, and the extra dose of collagen you'll add will make them even better for you.

My own current favorite green smoothie, by the way, is the Lemon Ginger Green Smoothie recipe on page 147. But every recipe is awesome, so pick any of them that tickle your fancy. Just be sure to rotate several different recipes so you'll get the wide range of phytochemicals you want.

Also, here are a few tips if you're new to making green smoothies:

- You can make your smoothies the night before. They'll keep for up to two days in the fridge; just make sure to cover them tightly. If they separate, pop them back into the blender for 10 to 20 seconds to recombine the ingredients.

- Remove the stems from collard greens, kale, and other veggies with tough stems.
- Blend your smoothies well. It can take a minute or more to get all the lumps out.
- Carefully measure the amounts of fruit and starchy veggies you use. Going overboard will make your smoothies too sugary.
- If you're new to green smoothies, or you're not a huge fan of greens, start with a recipe that features spinach rather than a more assertive green. Spinach is very mild, and you'll hardly even notice it.

Be sure to use a high-quality protein. Dr. Kellyann's Collagen Shakes and Bone Broth Protein, both available on my website, are great choices.

If you're already a pro at green smoothies, you can have fun creating your own recipes. Simply follow this formula:

Build-It-Yourself Green Smoothie

Prep time: 3 min. • Yield: 1 serving

1 to 2 scoops collagen protein powder (15 to 25 grams protein)

1 serving fat (page 57)

2 handfuls of leafy greens or non-starchy veggies (pages 55 and 56)

½ cup fruit or starchy veggies (pages 55 and 56)

Stevia or monk fruit sweetener to taste (optional)

Herbs and spices to taste (optional)

1 cup water, coconut milk (not canned), or almond milk, unsweetened and carrageenan-free

If you're new to smoothies, on the other hand, try my delicious, super-easy, tried-and-true recipes. You'll find everything from sweet, fruity smoothies to savory versions. (You'll be crazy about these savory smoothies if you're a fan of gazpacho and other cold vegetable soups.) I hope you love them all . . . *bon appétit!*

Apple Ginger Green Smoothie

Prep time: 3 min. • Yield: 1 serving

1 cup water, coconut milk (not canned), or almond milk, unsweetened and carrageenan-free

1/4 avocado

1 packet Dr. Kellyann's Vanilla Collagen Shake or 1 scoop Dr. Kellyann's Vanilla Bone Broth Protein (or 15 to 25 grams of high-quality vanilla collagen protein powder)

1/2 medium apple, diced

1 Persian cucumber or 3- to 4-inch piece English cucumber, sliced (about 1/2 cup after slicing)

1/4-inch piece fresh ginger, peeled and sliced

Pinch of ground cinnamon

2 handfuls (about 1 cup) of baby spinach, chopped

Pinch of Celtic or pink Himalayan salt (optional)

Ice, add to blender or pour smoothie over ice (optional)

In a blender, combine the water, avocado, collagen powder, apple, cucumber, ginger, cinnamon, spinach, salt (if using), and ice (if using). Blend until smooth and creamy.

If the smoothie is too thick, add more water, coconut milk, or almond milk to reach the desired consistency.

Bloody Mary Smoothie

Prep time: 3 min. • Yield: 1 serving

1 cup water

Juice of ½ lime

1 Persian cucumber or 3- to 4-inch piece English cucumber, sliced (about ½ cup after slicing)

1 scoop or 1 packet Dr. Kellyann's Flavorless Collagen Protein (or 15 to 25 grams of high-quality flavorless collagen protein powder)

¼ avocado

1 or 2 celery stalks

6 to 8 sweet grape or cherry tomatoes or 1 Roma tomato, chopped

2 handfuls of kale, stems removed, chopped (about 1 cup)

Dash hot sauce or cayenne or ¼ to ½ jalapeño pepper, seeded

½ teaspoon coconut aminos

½ to 1 teaspoon prepared horseradish

Celtic or pink Himalayan salt and freshly ground black pepper to taste (optional)

Ice, add to blender or pour smoothie over ice (optional)

In a blender, combine the water, lime juice, cucumber, collagen protein, avocado, celery, tomatoes, kale, hot sauce, aminos, horseradish, salt and pepper (if using), and ice (if using). Blend until smooth and creamy.

If the smoothie is too thick, add more water to reach the desired consistency.

Carrot Cake Green Smoothie

Prep time: 3 min. • Yield: 1 serving

¼ cup water, coconut milk (not canned), or almond milk, unsweetened and carrageenan-free

⅓ cup canned full-fat coconut milk

1 packet Dr. Kellyann's Vanilla Collagen Shake or 1 scoop Dr. Kellyann's Vanilla Bone Broth Protein (or 15 to 25 grams of high-quality vanilla collagen protein powder)

½ small carrot (about a 3-inch piece), shredded

½ cup fresh, frozen, or canned unsweetened pineapple, cubed

Pinch of ground cinnamon

Pinch of ground nutmeg

2 handfuls (about 1 cup) of baby spinach, chopped

Ice, add to blender or pour smoothie over ice (optional)

In a blender, combine the water, canned coconut milk, collagen powder, carrot, pineapple, cinnamon, nutmeg, spinach, and ice (if using). Blend until smooth and creamy.

If the smoothie is too thick, add more water, coconut milk, or almond milk to reach the desired consistency.

Cool Watermelon Green Smoothie

Prep time: 3 min. • Yield: 1 serving

½ to 1 cup water, coconut milk (not canned), or almond milk, unsweetened and carrageenan-free

1 cup watermelon, cubed

1 Persian cucumber or 3- to 4-inch piece English cucumber, sliced (about ½ cup after slicing; optional)

1 packet Dr. Kellyann's Vanilla Collagen Shake, 1 scoop Dr. Kellyann's Vanilla Bone Broth Protein, or 1 scoop or packet Dr. Kellyann's Flavorless Collagen Protein (or 15 to 25 grams of high-quality vanilla or flavorless collagen protein powder)

1 tablespoon avocado or MCT oil or ⅓ cup canned full-fat coconut milk

2 handfuls (about 1 cup) of baby spinach, chopped

Stevia or monk fruit sweetener to taste (optional if using flavorless collagen)

Ice, add to blender or pour smoothie over ice (optional)

In a blender, combine the water, watermelon, cucumber, collagen powder, oil, spinach, stevia (if using), and ice (if using). Blend until smooth and creamy.

If the smoothie is too thick, add more water, coconut milk, or almond milk to reach the desired consistency.

Notes

If you prefer a creamy smoothie, use coconut or almond milk, vanilla protein powder, and canned coconut milk (instead of the oil).

If you prefer more of a slushy consistency, use water, flavorless collagen, and stevia or monk fruit sweetener.

Creamy Pumpkin Spice Green Smoothie

Prep time: 3 min. • Yield: 1 serving

¼ cup water, coconut milk (not canned), or almond milk, unsweetened and carrageenan-free

⅓ cup canned full-fat coconut milk

1 packet Dr. Kellyann's Vanilla Collagen Shake or 1 scoop Dr. Kellyann's Vanilla Bone Broth Protein (or 15 to 25 grams of high-quality vanilla collagen protein powder)

½ cup canned pumpkin (not pie filling)

¼- to ½-inch piece fresh ginger, peeled and grated

Pinch of ground nutmeg

Pinch of ground cinnamon

2 handfuls (about 1 cup) of baby spinach, chopped

Ice, add to blender or pour smoothie over ice (optional)

In a blender, combine the water, canned coconut milk, collagen powder, pumpkin, ginger, nutmeg, cinnamon, spinach, and ice (if using). Blend until smooth and creamy.

If the smoothie is too thick, add more water, coconut milk, or almond milk to reach the desired consistency.

Cucumber Melon Green Smoothie

Prep time: 3 min. • Yield: 1 serving

½ to 1 cup water

Juice of ½ lime

1 Persian cucumber or 3- to 4-inch piece English cucumber, sliced (about ½ cup after slicing)

1 cup honeydew melon, cubed

1 scoop or 1 packet Dr. Kellyann's Flavorless Collagen Protein (or 15 to 25 grams of high-quality flavorless collagen protein powder)

½-inch piece fresh ginger, peeled and grated

4 teaspoons chia seeds

5 or 6 fresh mint leaves

2 handfuls of kale, stems removed, chopped (about 1 cup)

Pinch of Celtic or pink Himalayan salt (optional)

Stevia or monk fruit sweetener to taste (optional)

Ice, add to blender or pour smoothie over ice (optional)

In a blender, combine the water, lime juice, cucumber, honeydew, collagen protein, ginger, chia seeds, mint, kale, salt (if using), stevia (if using), and ice (if using). Blend until smooth and creamy.

If the smoothie is too thick, add more water to reach the desired consistency.

Note

Chia seeds will thicken the smoothie as it sits. If you don't like that consistency, select another fat from the approved list such as ¼ avocado or 1 tablespoon MCT oil.

Lemon Ginger Green Smoothie

Prep time: 3 min. • Yield: 1 serving

1 cup water

Juice of ½ lemon

1 teaspoon lemon zest

1 tablespoon avocado or olive oil

1 Persian cucumber or 3- to 4-inch piece English cucumber, sliced (about ½ cup after slicing)

1 scoop or 1 packet Dr. Kellyann's Flavorless Collagen Protein (or 15 to 25 grams of high-quality flavorless collagen protein powder)

½-inch piece fresh ginger, peeled and grated

2 handfuls (about 1 cup) of baby spinach, chopped

Stevia or monk fruit sweetener to taste (optional)

Ice, add to blender or pour smoothie over ice (optional)

In a blender, combine the water, lemon juice, lemon zest, oil, cucumber, collagen protein, ginger, spinach, stevia (if using), and ice (if using). Blend until smooth and creamy.

If the smoothie is too thick, add more water to reach the desired consistency.

Mexican Fiesta Green Smoothie

Prep time: 3 min. • Yield: 1 serving

1 cup water

Juice of ½ lime

1 scoop or 1 packet Dr. Kellyann's Flavorless Collagen Protein (or 15 to 25 grams of high-quality flavorless collagen protein powder)

¼ avocado

1 small tomatillo, chopped

1 small handful of cilantro (about ½ cup)

2 handfuls of rainbow or green Swiss chard, stems removed, chopped (about 1 cup)

Pinch of dried oregano

Pinch of cayenne pepper

Pinch of garlic powder (optional)

Celtic or pink Himalayan salt and freshly ground black pepper to taste (optional)

Ice, add to blender or pour smoothie over ice (optional)

In a blender, combine the water, lime juice, collagen protein, avocado, tomatillo, cilantro, chard, oregano, cayenne pepper, garlic powder (if using), salt and pepper (if using), and ice (if using). Blend until smooth and creamy.

If the smoothie is too thick, add more water to reach the desired consistency.

Papaya Ginger Green Smoothie

Prep time: 3 min. • Yield: 1 serving

1 cup water, coconut milk (not canned), or almond milk, unsweetened and carrageenan-free

Juice of ½ lemon (if using flavorless collagen)

¼ avocado or ⅓ cup canned full-fat coconut milk

1 packet Dr. Kellyann's Vanilla Collagen Shake, 1 scoop Dr. Kellyann's Vanilla Bone Broth Protein, or 1 scoop or packet Dr. Kellyann's Flavorless Collagen Protein (or 15 to 25 grams of high-quality vanilla or flavorless collagen protein powder)

1 cup fresh or frozen papaya, cubed

½-inch piece fresh ginger, peeled and grated

Pinch of ground nutmeg

Pinch of ground allspice (optional)

2 handfuls of kale, stems removed, chopped (about 1 cup)

Stevia or monk fruit sweetener to taste (optional if using flavorless collagen)

Ice, add to blender or pour smoothie over ice (optional)

In a blender, combine the water, lemon juice (if using), avocado, collagen powder, papaya, ginger, nutmeg, allspice (if using), kale, stevia (if using), and ice (if using). Blend until smooth and creamy.

If the smoothie is too thick, add more water, coconut milk, or almond milk to reached the desired consistency.

Notes

Papaya will congeal and thicken the smoothie, so it's best to drink it right after making it.

If you prefer a creamy smoothie, use almond or coconut milk, vanilla protein powder, and canned coconut milk.

If you prefer more of a slushy consistency, use water, lemon, flavorless collagen, and stevia or monk fruit sweetener.

Pineapple Mint Green Smoothie

Prep time: 3 min. • Yield: 1 serving

½ to 1 cup water, coconut milk (not canned), or almond milk, unsweetened and carrageenan-free

Juice of ½ lemon (if using flavorless collagen)

¼ avocado or ⅓ cup canned full-fat coconut milk

1 packet Dr. Kellyann's Vanilla Collagen Shake, 1 scoop Dr. Kellyann's Vanilla Bone Broth Protein, or 1 scoop or packet Dr. Kellyann's Flavorless Collagen Protein (or 15 to 25 grams of high-quality vanilla or flavorless collagen protein powder)

1 cup fresh, frozen, or canned unsweetened pineapple chunks

5 to 6 fresh mint leaves

½-inch piece fresh ginger, peeled and grated (optional)

2 handfuls (about 1 cup) of baby spinach, chopped

Stevia or monk fruit sweetener to taste (optional if using flavorless collagen)

Ice, add to blender or pour smoothie over ice (optional)

In a blender, combine the water, lemon juice (if using), avocado, collagen powder, pineapple, mint, ginger (if using), spinach, stevia (if using), and ice (if using). Blend until smooth and creamy.

If the smoothie is too thick, add more water, coconut milk, or almond milk to reach the desired consistency.

Notes

If you prefer a creamy smoothie, use ⅓ cup coconut or almond milk, vanilla protein powder, and canned coconut milk.

If you prefer more of a slushy consistency, use 1 cup water, lemon juice, avocado, flavorless collagen, and stevia or monk fruit sweetener.

Savory Mediterranean Green Smoothie

Prep time: 3 min. • Yield: 1 serving

1 cup water

Juice of ½ lemon

1 scoop or 1 packet Dr. Kellyann's Flavorless Collagen Protein (or 15 to 25 grams of high-quality flavorless collagen protein powder)

2 teaspoons olive oil

4 to 5 kalamata or green olives, pitted

1 Persian cucumber or 3- to 4-inch piece English cucumber, sliced (about ½ cup)

1 to 2 tablespoons fresh dill or basil

1 handful of arugula, chopped (about ½ cup)

1 handful of lettuce or baby spinach, chopped (about ½ cup)

Freshly ground black pepper to taste (optional)

Dash hot sauce (optional)

Ice, add to blender or pour smoothie over ice (optional)

In a blender, combine the water, lemon juice, collagen protein, oil, olives, cucumber, dill, arugula, lettuce, pepper (if using), hot sauce (if using), and ice (if using). Blend until smooth and creamy.

If the smoothie is too thick, add more water to reach the desired consistency.

Savory Salad Bowl Smoothie

Prep time: 3 min. • Yield: 1 serving

1 cup water

Juice of ½ lemon

¼ avocado

1 scoop or 1 packet Dr. Kellyann's Flavorless Collagen Protein (or 15 to 25 grams of high-quality flavorless collagen protein powder)

1 Persian cucumber or 3- to 4-inch piece English cucumber, sliced (about ½ cup)

1 celery stalk, chopped

6 grape or cherry tomatoes or 1 Roma tomato, chopped

1 small handful (about ½ cup) of Italian parsley

4 romaine leaves, chopped

Pinch of Italian seasoning

Celtic or pink Himalayan salt and freshly ground black pepper to taste (optional)

Ice, add to blender or pour smoothie over ice (optional)

In a blender, combine the water, lemon juice, avocado, collagen protein, cucumber, celery, tomatoes, parlsey, romaine, Italian seasoning, salt and pepper (if using), and ice (if using). Blend until smooth.

If the smoothie is too thick, add more water to reach the desired consistency.

Savory Tomato Basil Smoothie

Prep time: 3 min. • Yield: 1 serving

1 cup water

Juice of ½ lime

1 scoop or 1 packet Dr. Kellyann's Flavorless Collagen Protein (or 15 to 25 grams of high-quality flavorless collagen protein powder)

1 tablespoon avocado or olive oil

1 Persian cucumber or 3- to 4-inch piece English cucumber, sliced (about ½ cup)

6 to 8 sweet grape or cherry tomatoes or 1 Roma tomato, chopped

1 small handful (about ½ cup) of basil, stems removed

4 or 5 butter lettuce leaves

Celtic or pink Himalayan salt and freshly ground black pepper to taste (optional)

Dash hot sauce or cayenne (optional)

Ice, add to blender or pour smoothie over ice (optional)

In a blender, combine the water, lime juice, collagen protein, oil, cucumber, tomatoes, basil, lettuce, salt and pepper (if using), hot sauce (if using), and ice (if using). Blend until smooth and creamy.

If the smoothie is too thick, add more water to reach the desired consistency.

Strawberry Green Smoothie

Prep time: 3 min. • Yield: 1 serving

½ to 1 cup water, coconut milk (not canned), or almond milk, unsweetened and carrageenan-free

Juice of ½ lemon (if using flavorless collagen)

1 cup fresh or frozen strawberries

1 packet Dr. Kellyann's Vanilla Collagen Shake, 1 scoop Dr. Kellyann's Vanilla Bone Broth Protein, or 1 scoop or 1 packet Dr. Kellyann's Flavorless Collagen Protein (or 15 to 25 grams of high-quality vanilla or flavorless collagen protein powder)

¼ avocado or ⅓ cup canned full-fat coconut milk

Stevia or monk fruit sweetener to taste (optional if using flavorless collagen)

3 or 4 romaine leaves, chopped (about 1 cup)

Ice, add to blender or pour smoothie over ice (optional)

In a blender, combine the water, lemon juice (if using), strawberries, collagen powder, avocado, stevia (if using), romaine, and ice (if using). Blend until smooth and creamy.

If the smoothie is too thick, add more water to reach the desired consistency.

Notes

If you prefer a creamy smoothie, use ½ cup coconut or almond milk, vanilla protein powder, and canned coconut milk.

If you prefer more of a slushy consistency, use 1 cup water, lemon juice, avocado, flavorless collagen, and stevia or monk fruit sweetener.

Vitamin C Boost Green Smoothie

Prep time: 3 min. • Yield: 1 serving

1 cup water

Juice of ½ lime or lemon

1 scoop or 1 packet Dr. Kellyann's Flavorless Collagen Protein (or 15 to 25 grams of high-quality flavorless collagen protein powder)

¼ avocado

½ cup strawberries

1 kiwi, peeled

½-inch piece fresh ginger, peeled and grated

2 handfuls of kale, stems removed, chopped (about 1 cup)

Stevia or monk fruit sweetener, to equal about 2 teaspoons sugar (optional)

Ice, add to blender or pour smoothie over ice (optional)

In a blender, combine the water, lime juice, collagen protein, avocado, strawberries, kiwi, ginger, kale, stevia (if using), and ice (if using). Blend until smooth and creamy.

If the smoothie is too thick, add more water to reach the desired consistency.

How to Make Green Smoothie Popsicles

Any of my green smoothies can be transformed into Popsicles if you want an icy treat on a hot day. This is a great healthy snack to keep on hand when you're on your lifestyle plan. (You can also turn your smoothies into Popsicles on your cleanse, but only if you're a real Popsicle lover and can eat several at one sitting!) Simply pour your smoothie into Popsicle molds or into 3-ounce paper cups and freeze until firm, or about 2 hours. The smoothies are large, and you will get several Popsicles from each smoothie.

If you're using paper cups or Popsicle molds without plastic handles, freeze for about 15 or 20 minutes before inserting wooden Popsicle sticks so they will stand upright.

Chapter 8

Rich, Creamy Shakes

Who doesn't love a cool, creamy, refreshing shake? That's why every day on this cleanse, you'll get to enjoy a delicious, filling shake for lunch. It's a sweet treat that's guilt-free because it's going to cleanse your cells and reinvigorate your body.

No matter what flavors are your favorites, you'll find something you love here, from decadent Chocolate Banana Walnut to exotic Tropical Pineapple Berry. Each shake is loaded with collagen, healthy fat, and nutrient-rich fruits or veggies.

If you're doing a keto-friendly cleanse, stick to shakes with non-starchy veggies and very-low-carb fruits like berries; otherwise, you can pick recipes that feature higher-carb fruits or starchy veggies. If you want to ramp up the nutritional power of any of my fruit-only shakes, just toss in a handful or two of spinach, kale, or chard.

Want to invent your own shakes? That's fine, too! Simply follow this formula and you're good to go:

Build-It-Yourself Shake

Prep time: 3 min. • Yield: 1 serving

1 to 2 scoops collagen protein powder (15 to 25 grams protein)

1 serving fat (page 57)

½ cup fruit or starchy veggie (pages 55 and 56)
(skip if doing the keto modification)

Stevia or monk fruit sweetener to taste (optional)

Herbs and spices to taste (optional)

1 cup water, coconut milk (not canned), or almond milk,
unsweetened and carrageenan-free

P.S.—If you create something absolutely fabulous, share it with us on my Facebook page at facebook.com/groups/DrKellyannsCleanseandReset/!

Chocolate Banana Walnut Shake

Prep time: 3 min. • Yield: 1 serving

1 cup water, coconut milk (not canned), or almond milk, unsweetened and carrageenan-free

½ medium banana (optionally frozen for a creamier shake)

1 packet Dr. Kellyann's Chocolate Collagen Shake or 1 scoop Dr. Kellyann's Chocolate Bone Broth Protein (or 15 to 25 grams of high-quality chocolate collagen protein powder)

1 tablespoon walnut oil or 2 tablespoons chopped walnuts

Ice, add to blender or pour shake over ice (optional)

In a blender, combine the water, banana, collagen powder, walnut oil, and ice (if using). Blend well.

Orange Blueberry Shake

Prep time: 3 min. • Yield: 1 serving

1 cup water, coconut milk
(not canned), or almond
milk, unsweetened and
carrageenan-free

2/3 cup blueberries (optionally
frozen for a creamier shake)

1 packet Dr. Kellyann's Collagen
Cooler, orange cream flavor

1/3 cup canned full-fat coconut milk

Ice, add to blender or pour
shake over ice (optional)

In a blender, combine the water, blueberries, collagen powder, canned coconut milk, and ice (if using). Blend well.

Tropical Pineapple Berry Shake

Prep time: 3 min. • Yield: 1 serving

1 cup water, coconut milk
(not canned), or almond
milk, unsweetened and
carrageenan-free

1/2 cup fresh, frozen, or canned
unsweetened pineapple (use
frozen for a creamier shake)

1/2 cup fresh or frozen strawberries

1 packet Dr. Kellyann's Vanilla
Collagen Shake, 1 scoop
Dr. Kellyann's Vanilla Bone Broth
Protein, or 1 scoop or packet
Dr. Kellyann's Flavorless Collagen
Protein (or 15 to 25 grams of
high-quality vanilla or flavorless
collagen protein powder)

1/3 cup canned full-fat coconut milk

1/2 teaspoon vanilla (if using
flavorless collagen)

Stevia or monk fruit sweetener
to equal 2 to 3 teaspoons
sugar (optional if using
flavorless collagen)

Ice, add to blender or pour
shake over ice (optional)

In a blender, combine the water, pineapple, strawberries, collagen powder, canned coconut milk, vanilla (if using), stevia (if using), and ice (if using). Blend well.

Why Is Whey Protein on the "No" List?

I know that whey protein is popular these days, but I want you to avoid it on your cleanse. Instead, use beef protein, or—if you're following the vegetarian, vegan, or pescatarian modifications (see pages 68 and 69)—use egg protein, pea protein, or marine collagen. Here's why.

Whey is the liquid that remains when milk is curdled and strained to make cheese. Many people think that eating whey is okay on a dairy-free diet because it doesn't contain casein, the milk protein that's most likely to cause sensitivity. But casein is only one potential troublemaker in whey protein.

There are three forms of whey protein: *whey protein concentrate, whey protein isolate,* and *whey protein hydrolysate*. Whey protein concentrate contains significant amounts of the milk sugar lactose, which can cause gas, bloating, and diarrhea. Whey protein isolate and whey protein hydrolysate, which are more highly refined products, are nearly or entirely lactose-free—but they can still cause GI problems because many people are allergic to whey itself. In fact, whey is the second most allergenic protein in milk.

In addition to its potential to be allergenic, whey protein powder often has added thickeners. These, too, can cause gas and cramping.

Once you're done with your cleanse, you can experiment with adding whey protein into your diet. Try it for three or four days and see if you tolerate it well or have a bad reaction.

Green Apple Ginger Shake

Prep time: 3 min. • Yield: 1 serving

1 cup water, coconut milk (not canned), or almond milk, unsweetened and carrageenan-free

⅓ cup canned full-fat coconut milk

½ tart green apple

½-inch piece fresh ginger, peeled and grated

1 packet Dr. Kellyann's Vanilla Collagen Shake, 1 scoop Dr. Kellyann's Vanilla Bone Broth Protein, or 1 scoop or packet Dr. Kellyann's Flavorless Collagen Protein (or 15 to 25 grams of high-quality vanilla or flavorless collagen protein powder)

Stevia or monk fruit sweetener (optional if using flavorless collagen)

Ice, add to blender or pour shake over ice (optional)

Pinch of ground cinnamon, for garnish (optional)

In a blender, combine the water, canned coconut milk, apple, ginger, collagen powder, stevia (if using), and ice (if using). Blend well. Garnish with a pinch of cinnamon, if desired.

Ginger Mango Shake

Prep time: 3 min. • Yield: 1 serving

1 cup water, coconut milk
(not canned), or almond
milk, unsweetened and
carrageenan-free

⅓ cup canned full-fat coconut milk

⅓ cup fresh or frozen mango

½-inch piece fresh ginger,
peeled and grated

1 packet Dr. Kellyann's Vanilla
Collagen Shake, 1 scoop
Dr. Kellyann's Vanilla Bone Broth
Protein, or 1 scoop or packet
Dr. Kellyann's Flavorless Collagen
Protein (or 15 to 25 grams of
high-quality vanilla or flavorless
collagen protein powder)

Stevia or monk fruit
sweetener (optional if using
flavorless collagen)

Ice, add to blender or pour
shake over ice (optional)

In a blender, combine the water, canned coconut milk, mango, ginger, collagen powder, stevia (if using), and ice (if using). Blend well.

Peachy Almond Shake

Prep time: 3 min. • Yield: 1 serving

1 cup water, coconut milk (not canned), or almond milk, unsweetened and carrageenan-free

1 tablespoon almond butter or 2 tablespoons almonds

1 or 2 drops natural almond extract (if using flavorless collagen)

1 peach, pitted and sliced (optional 1 slice reserved for garnish)

1 packet Dr. Kellyann's Vanilla Collagen Shake, 1 scoop Dr. Kellyann's Vanilla Bone Broth Protein, or 1 scoop or packet Dr. Kellyann's Flavorless Collagen Protein (or 15 to 25 grams of high-quality vanilla or flavorless collagen protein powder)

Stevia or monk fruit sweetener (optional if using flavorless collagen)

Ice, add to blender or pour shake over ice (optional)

Pinch of ground nutmeg, for garnish (optional)

In a blender, combine the water, almond butter, almond extract (if using), peach, collagen powder, stevia (if using), and ice (if using). Blend well. Garnish with a fresh peach slice or a pinch of nutmeg, if desired.

Piña Colada Shake

Prep time: 3 min. • Yield: 1 serving

1 cup water, coconut milk (not canned), or almond milk, unsweetened and carrageenan-free

⅓ cup canned full-fat coconut milk

½ cup fresh, frozen, or canned unsweetened pineapple

1 packet Dr. Kellyann's Vanilla Collagen Shake, 1 scoop Dr. Kellyann's Vanilla Bone Broth Protein, or 1 scoop or packet Dr. Kellyann's Flavorless Collagen Protein (or 15 to 25 grams of high-quality vanilla or flavorless collagen protein powder)

Stevia or monk fruit sweetener (optional if using flavorless collagen)

Ice, add to blender or pour shake over ice (optional)

In a blender, combine the water, canned coconut milk, pineapple, collagen powder, stevia (if using), and ice (if using). Blend well.

Peachy Strawberry Shake

Prep time: 3 min. • Yield: 1 serving

1 cup water, coconut milk (not canned), or almond milk, unsweetened and carrageenan-free

⅓ cup canned full-fat coconut milk

½ cup of fresh or frozen strawberries

1 small peach, pitted and sliced

½ to 1 teaspoon pure vanilla extract (optional if using flavorless collagen)

1 packet Dr. Kellyann's Vanilla Collagen Shake, 1 scoop Dr. Kellyann's Vanilla Bone Broth Protein, or 1 scoop or packet Dr. Kellyann's Flavorless Collagen Protein (or 15 to 25 grams of high-quality vanilla or flavorless collagen protein powder)

Stevia or monk fruit sweetener (optional if using flavorless collagen)

Ice, add to blender or pour shake over ice (optional)

In a blender, combine the water, canned coconut milk, strawberries, peach, vanilla (if using), collagen powder, stevia (if using), and ice (if using). Blend well.

Berries and Cream Shake

Prep time: 3 min. • Yield: 1 serving

1 cup water, coconut milk (not canned), or almond milk, unsweetened and carrageenan-free

⅓ cup canned full-fat coconut milk

½ cup assorted berries (strawberries, blueberries, raspberries, blackberries, or mixed berries)

½ teaspoon pure vanilla extract (if using flavorless collagen)

1 packet Dr. Kellyann's Vanilla Collagen Shake, 1 scoop Dr. Kellyann's Vanilla Bone Broth Protein, or 1 scoop or packet Dr. Kellyann's Flavorless Collagen Protein (or 15 to 25 grams of high-quality vanilla or flavorless collagen protein powder)

Stevia or monk fruit sweetener (optional if using flavorless collagen)

Ice, add to blender or pour shake over ice (optional)

In a blender, combine the water, canned coconut milk, berries, vanilla (if using), collagen powder, stevia (if using), and ice (if using). Blend well.

Supercharged Chocolate Shake

Prep time: 3 min. • Yield: 1 serving

1 cup water, coconut milk (not canned), or almond milk, unsweetened and carrageenan-free

1 cup fresh spinach

1/2 cup blueberries

1 tablespoon ground flaxseed or hemp seeds

1/4 avocado

1 packet Dr. Kellyann's Chocolate Collagen Shake or 1 scoop Dr. Kellyann's Chocolate Bone Broth Protein (or 15 to 25 grams of high-quality chocolate or flavorless collagen protein powder)

Ice, add to blender or pour shake over ice (optional)

In a blender, combine the water, spinach, blueberries, flaxseed, avocado, collagen powder, and ice (if using). Blend well.

Black Cherry Almond Shake

Prep time: 3 min. • Yield: 1 serving

1 cup water, coconut milk (not canned), or almond milk, unsweetened and carrageenan-free

1/3 cup canned full-fat coconut milk

1/2 cup frozen black cherries

1 to 2 drops natural almond extract (if using flavorless collagen)

1 packet Dr. Kellyann's Vanilla or Chocolate Collagen Shake, 1 scoop Dr. Kellyann's Vanilla or Chocolate Bone Broth Protein, or 1 scoop or packet Dr. Kellyann's Flavorless Collagen Protein (or 15 to 25 grams of high-quality chocolate, vanilla, or flavorless collagen protein powder)

Stevia or monk fruit sweetener (optional if using flavorless collagen)

Ice, add to blender or pour shake over ice (optional)

In a blender, combine the water, canned coconut milk, cherries, almond extract, collagen powder, stevia (if using), and ice (if using). Blend well.

Lemon Cream Shake

Prep time: 3 min. • Yield: 1 serving

1 cup water, coconut milk (not canned), or almond milk, unsweetened and carrageenan-free

⅓ cup canned full-fat coconut milk

1 or 2 drops natural lemon extract

1 teaspoon fresh lemon juice

1 packet Dr. Kellyann's Vanilla Collagen Shake, 1 scoop Dr. Kellyann's Vanilla Bone Broth Protein, or 1 scoop or packet Dr. Kellyann's Flavorless Collagen Protein (or 15 to 25 grams of high-quality vanilla or flavorless collagen protein powder)

Stevia or monk fruit sweetener (optional if using flavorless collagen)

Ice, add to blender or pour shake over ice (optional)

Pinch of lemon zest, for garnish (optional)

In a blender, combine the water, canned coconut milk, lemon extract, lemon juice, collagen powder, stevia (if using), and ice (if using). Blend well. Garnish with a little lemon zest, if desired.

You may notice in my recipes that when I offer almond milk as an option, I ask you to make sure that it's carrageenan-free. (Same for coconut milk.) Here's why.

Carrageenan is an emulsifier that manufacturers add to almond milk so you don't need to shake the carton to blend the contents. It's made from red algae or seaweed, so you'd expect it to be good for you—but it's not. In fact, it's very, very bad news.

Researcher Joanne Tobacman, who's studied carrageenan for years, has lobbied the government to ban it as a food additive. Her research implicates carrageenan as a culprit in gastrointestinal malignancy[1] and breast cancer.[2] In addition, her studies indicate that carrageenan may contribute to glucose intolerance and insulin insensitivity,[3] both of which are steps on the road to diabetes.

Moreover, Tobacman isn't talking about massive doses of carrageenan. In fact, the mice in her diabetes research consume *less* carrageenan per body weight than the average American. What's more, she's using the same food-grade form that manufacturers use.

In short, even small doses of carrageenan may inflame your body and put you at higher risk for cancer or diabetes. Does that sound like something you want in your diet? Nope.

Now that you know the bad news, let's get back to the good news. If you read labels carefully, you can find brands of coconut milk and almond milk that don't contain carrageenan, sugar, or other unnecessary ingredients.

Better yet, there's a simple solution, at least when it comes to almond milk: make your own at home! It's fun, it's easy, and you'll wind up with a milk that has no additives and contains more protein than the store-bought variety.

Making your own almond milk takes just a few minutes of actual work. (The rest is soaking time.) Here's how to do it.

Make-It-Yourself Almond Milk

Prep time: 10 min. • Yield: about 5 cups

1½ cups whole raw almonds, optionally blanched

4 cups purified water for almond milk, plus more for
    soaking

1 teaspoon pure vanilla extract

Place the almonds in a medium bowl. Cover with the water and let the nuts soak for at least 4 hours, or up to 2 days for creamier almond milk.

Drain the water and place the almonds in a blender. Add 2 cups of the water and blend to a creamy paste. Add the other 2 cups of water and the vanilla. Blend for 3 to 4 minutes.

Strain the almond milk in a fine-mesh sieve lined with cheesecloth or in a nut bag. Drain all the milk from the solids. Refrigerate. Store in a sealed container in the refrigerator for up to 3 days.

Apple Pie Shake

Prep time: 5 min. • Yield: 1 serving

1 cup water, coconut milk (not canned), or almond milk, unsweetened and carrageenan-free

⅓ cup canned full-fat coconut milk

1 small apple, cored and sliced

1 teaspoon pure vanilla extract (if using flavorless collagen)

¼ teaspoon ground cinnamon, plus more for garnish

Pinch of ground nutmeg, plus more for garnish

1 packet Dr. Kellyann's Vanilla Collagen Shake, 1 scoop Dr. Kellyann's Vanilla Bone Broth Protein, or 1 scoop or packet Dr. Kellyann's Flavorless Collagen Protein (or 15 to 25 grams of high-quality vanilla or flavorless collagen protein powder)

Stevia or monk fruit sweetener (optional if using flavorless collagen)

Ice, add to blender or pour shake over ice (optional)

In a blender, combine the water, canned coconut milk, apple, vanilla (if using), cinnamon, nutmeg, collagen powder, stevia (if using), and ice (if using). Blend well. Garnish with additional cinnamon or nutmeg, if desired.

Chocolate Raspberry Shake

Prep time: 3 min. • Yield: 1 serving

1 cup water, coconut milk (not canned), or almond milk, unsweetened and carrageenan-free

⅓ cup canned full-fat coconut milk

½ cup raspberries, plus more for garnish

1 packet Dr. Kellyann's Chocolate Collagen Shake or 1 scoop Dr. Kellyann's Chocolate Bone Broth Protein (or 15 to 25 grams of high-quality chocolate collagen protein powder)

Ice, add to blender or pour shake over ice (optional)

In a blender, combine the water, canned coconut milk, raspberries, collagen powder, and ice (if using). Blend well. Garnish with a few raspberries, if desired.

Orange Creamsicle Shake

Prep time: 3 min. • Yield: 1 serving

1 cup water, coconut milk
(not canned) or almond
milk, unsweetened and
carrageenan-free

⅓ cup canned full-fat coconut milk

1 small orange, peeled and
seeds removed

1 packet Dr. Kellyann's Vanilla
Collagen Shake, 1 scoop
Dr. Kellyann's Vanilla Bone Broth
Protein, or 1 scoop or packet
Dr. Kellyann's Flavorless Collagen
Protein (or 15 to 25 grams of
high-quality vanilla or flavorless
collagen protein powder)

Stevia or monk fruit
sweetener (optional if using
flavorless collagen)

Ice, add to blender or pour
shake over ice (optional)

In a blender, combine the water, canned coconut milk, orange, collagen powder, stevia (if using), and ice (if using). Blend well.

Chapter 9

Beautiful Broth
Loading Soups

B roth loading soups are a centerpiece of this cleanse, and you're
going to love them. That's because they're warm, comforting, and
nourishing, and they'll help you relax and unwind after a long day.

I call these soul-soothing soups "broth loading" because they're
going to load you up with all of the nutrients in bone broth, plus
healthy fats and nutrient-packed veggies. As a result, they're going to
do everything from strengthening your gut wall to removing toxins
to beautifying your skin and making your eyes sparkle. What's more,
these soups will make your evenings craving-free because they're so
filling that they'll keep you satisfied for hours and hours.

Now, here's a tip for eating your soup: savor it slowly! Eating slowly
and mindfully allows you to enjoy your food more, and research shows
that it makes you feel full longer—which may explain why eating
slowly is linked to having a smaller body mass.[1]

So light a candle, serve your soup in a fancy bowl, and appreciate
each delicious bite. This is a perfect time to slow your life down and let
go of a day's worth of stress. The saying is true: Soup is food not just
for the body but also for the soul.

By the way, if you want to create your own soups, that's great! Just follow this "recipe":

Build-It-Yourself Soup

Prep time: 5 min. • Cook time: 5 min. • Yield: 1-2 servings

2 cups prepared broth

1 serving healthy fat (page 57)

2 cups leafy greens or non-starchy veggies (pages 55 and 56)

½ cup starchy veggie (pages 55 and 56; skip if doing the keto modification)

Herbs and spices to taste (optional)

If you decide to invent your own recipes, here are some tips for creating flavor-packed soups using herbs or spices:

- Thyme works well in a creamy soup like cauliflower or mushroom soup.
- Try Italian seasonings like basil, oregano, and thyme in a creamy tomato soup.
- Make a Mexican-style soup with cumin, chili powder, and paprika.
- Dill, parsley, and lemon zest are delicious in a chilled cucumber soup.
- If you're adding herbs and spices to 8 to 16 ounces of bone broth, start by adding a shake or two of each herb or spice and then season to taste. If you're making larger batches of a broth loading soup (32 ounces or more), start with ½ teaspoon of each herb and spice you want to add, and then taste-test and season to your liking.

Whether you choose one of my recipes or create one of your own, the foundation of your soup will be a beautiful bone broth. Here are some of my best tips for making it (along with Instant Pot directions).

Once your cleanse is done and you're on Dr. Kellyann's Lifestyle Plan, you can turn many of my soup recipes into meals simply by adding meat. It's a great way to eat healthy and stretch the family budget. I've added notes to these recipes suggesting which meats you can add to them post-cleanse.

Tips on Making Your Bone Broth

If you're buying your bone broth in the store or online (Dr. Kellyann's Chicken and Bone Broths, available at DrKellyann.com, are a good option), you can skip this section. But if you're new to bone broth and are planning on making your own, I have a few words of advice for you.

The first thing I want to say is: relax! Nothing is simpler than making your own bone broth. After all, the earliest humans made bone broth in animal skins over a fire, which tells you that it doesn't require a lot of finesse. So don't worry—you've got this.

While your broth will be wonderful even if it's perfectly imperfect, here are a few tips for getting the best results:

- Buy collagen-rich bones. For beef, go with knuckle bones, joint bones, or marrow bones if you can get them. For chicken, go with a whole carcass, legs, wings, necks, and backs. If you aren't sure which bones to get, ask your butcher to help you out. If you have leftover bones from dinners, save them and toss them in as well. (I also like to add some bones with meat on them, to give my broth a richer flavor.) Bones can go into your broth either preroasted or raw.

- Let your broth simmer slowly over low heat. Be sure to cook it for at least the minimum amount of time stated in the recipe.
- Add just enough water to keep your ingredients covered. This will give you a rich, full-flavored broth.
- Package your broth in small containers and store it in the freezer. That way, it'll stay fresh and thaw quickly when you want to use it.

Your broth should be jiggly when you chill it, because that means it's loaded with gelatin. However, even non-jiggly broth has lots of gelatin in it, and it'll do the trick. (A few troubleshooting tips to get more jiggle next time: stick close to the cooking times above, and make sure your broth simmers rather than boils. Also, ask your butcher to select cartilage-rich bones for you.) If you want to give your broth even more jiggle, you can always add a packet of collagen powder.

Finally, don't fret if you're missing ingredients or want to leave some out. Here are some tips:

- Out of vinegar? The vinegar helps to pull more nutrients out of the bones—but if you don't have any, you can use lemon juice or no acid at all.
- Don't have the spices the recipe calls for? Substitute any spices you like.
- Don't like garlic? Add less, or none at all. Love garlic? Feel free to add more.
- Using meaty bones and can't afford grass-fed beef or organic chicken? Simply remove the extra fat on the beef or the skin on the chicken and you're good to go.
- Allergic to any of the veggies (or hate them)? No problem—just leave them out.

As you can see, in addition to being easy to make, bone broth is adaptable . . . so have fun putting your own personal stamp on your batches.

How to Make Your Broth in an Instant Pot

If you're busy and don't have time to watch over a pot of bone broth, I have an easy solution for you: make your broth in an Instant Pot! Here are some tips for creating Instant Pot broth.

Cooking on both high and low pressure can result in a rich, gelatinous broth. However, if you have the extra time, low-pressure cooking may give you better and more consistent results.

The length of time required for making bone broth in an Instant Pot depends on several factors, including which pressure setting you select as well as the type and quantity of bones you're using. However, for a six-quart Instant Pot on high pressure, chicken bone broth typically takes ninety minutes while beef bone broth usually requires two hours. For low pressure cooking, chicken bone broth takes two hours and beef requires approximately three hours.

These times refer only to the actual pressure-cooking time. Allow for additional time:

- if you choose to first roast your beef bones (to enhance the flavor)
- for presoaking in apple cider vinegar
- for the Instant Pot to reach the appropriate pressure
- to naturally release the pressure at the end (this can take up to ninety minutes)

The whole process from start to finish typically takes four to six hours—which is still much faster than making broth in a slow cooker or on the stovetop. And if you're like me, every extra minute you can save in a day counts!

	POULTRY	BEEF	FISH
Stove/Slow Cooker	4 to 8 hours	12 to 24 hours	Not recommended
Instant Pot	1.5 to 2 hours on high; 2 to 3 hours on low	2 to 3 hours on high; 3 to 4 on low	Not recommended

Beef Bone Broth

Prep time: 15 min. • Cook time: 3 to 12 hours depending on cooking mode • Yield: 1 gallon of broth

3 or more pounds beef bones

2 or more pounds meaty bones, such as oxtail, short ribs, etc.

¼ cup apple cider vinegar

Purified water

2 ripe tomatoes, cut in wedges

2 to 4 carrots, scrubbed and roughly chopped

3 to 4 celery stalks, including leafy part, roughly chopped

1 medium onion, cut into large wedges

1 to 2 garlic cloves

2 bay leaves

2 teaspoons Celtic or pink Himalayan salt

1 teaspoon peppercorns

Fat-burning spices you can add for more fat-burning power:

1 tablespoon instant espresso powder

1-inch piece fresh ginger, sliced

Handful of parsley or cilantro

1 teaspoon fresh or ground turmeric

¹⁄₁₆ to ⅛ teaspoon cayenne

1-2 teaspoons ground cumin

Place all the bones into a large stockpot, slow cooker, or pressure cooker. Add the vinegar and enough purified water to cover everything by 1 inch. Add all the vegetables, herbs, and spices. Add more water, if necessary. Follow the instructions for the mode of cooking you choose.

On the stovetop on medium heat, bring the water to a simmer and reduce the heat to low. Cover and let simmer for at least 12 hours and up to 24. Add water as needed so the bones are always covered.

In a slow cooker, set to low, cover, and cook for at least 12 hours and up to 24 hours. Add water as needed so the bones are always covered.

In a pressure cooker or Instant Pot, using your cooker's instructions, bring up to full pressure. Reduce the heat to low, maintaining full pressure, and cook for 3 hours. Allow the pressure to naturally release.

When the broth is done, remove all the bones and meat and pour the broth through a fine-mesh strainer into a large bowl. Discard the solids and reserve the meat for another use. (You can also refrigerate or freeze the bones and reuse them to make more broth.)

Let the broth cool completely before covering and placing in the refrigerator. When chilled the broth should be very gelatinous.

The broth will keep for 5 days in the refrigerator and 3 or more months in the freezer.

Note

Joint, neck, and knuckle bones are best for making bone broth because they have the largest amount of collagen. Marrow bones are also excellent.

Chicken Bone Broth

Prep time: 15 min. • Cook time: 2 to 8 hours depending on cooking mode • Yield: 1 gallon of broth

3 or more pounds raw or cooked chicken bones or carcasses

2 or more pounds chicken thighs, legs, and/or wings

6 to 8 chicken feet (optional; they'll add a great deal of collagen to your broth)

1/4 cup apple cider vinegar

Purified water

2 to 4 carrots, scrubbed and roughly chopped

3 to 4 celery stalks, including leafy part, roughly chopped

1 medium onion, cut into large chunks

1 to 2 garlic cloves

1 bay leaf

2 teaspoons Celtic or pink Himalayan salt

1 teaspoon peppercorns

Fat-burning spices you can add for more fat-burning power:

1-inch piece fresh ginger, sliced

Handful of parsley or cilantro

1 teaspoon fresh or ground turmeric

1/16 to 1/8 teaspoon cayenne

1 to 2 teaspoons ground cumin

(recipe continues)

Place all the bones into a large stockpot, slow cooker, or pressure cooker. Add the vinegar and enough purified water to cover everything by 1 inch. Add all the vegetables, herbs, and spices. Add more water, if necessary. Follow the instructions for the mode of cooking you choose.

On the stovetop on medium heat, bring the water to a simmer and reduce the heat to low. Cover and let simmer for at least 4 hours and up to 8. Add water as needed so the bones are always covered.

In a slow cooker, set to low, cover, and cook for 8 hours.

In a pressure cooker or Instant Pot, using your cooker's instructions, bring up to full pressure. Reduce the heat to low, maintaining full pressure, and cook for 2 hours. Allow the pressure to naturally release.

When the broth is done, remove all the bones and the meat and pour the broth through a fine-mesh strainer into a large bowl. Discard the solids and reserve the meat for another use. (You can also refrigerate or freeze the bones and reuse them to make more broth.)

Let the broth cool completely before covering and placing into the refrigerator. When chilled the broth should be very gelatinous.

The broth will keep for 5 days in the refrigerator and 3 or more months in the freezer.

Rotisserie Chicken Bone Broth

Prep time: 15 min. • Cook time: 2 to 8 hours depending on cooking mode • Yield: 1 gallon of broth

3 or more carcasses from rotisserie chickens

Drumsticks, thighs and wings from a rotisserie chicken or 2 or more pounds chicken thighs, legs, and/or wings

6 to 8 chicken feet (optional; they'll add a great deal of collagen to your broth)

¼ cup apple cider vinegar

Purified water

2 to 4 carrots, scrubbed and roughly chopped

3 to 4 celery stalks, including leafy part, roughly chopped

1 medium onion, cut into large chunks

1 to 2 garlic cloves

1 bay leaf

2 teaspoons Celtic or pink Himalayan salt

1 teaspoon peppercorns

Fat-burning spices you can add for more fat-burning power:

1-inch piece fresh ginger, sliced

Handful of parsley or cilantro

1 teaspoon fresh or ground turmeric

$\frac{1}{16}$ to $\frac{1}{8}$ teaspoon cayenne

1 to 2 teaspoons ground cumin

Place all the bones into a large stockpot, slow cooker, or pressure cooker. Add the vinegar and enough purified water to cover everything by 1 inch. Add all the vegetables, herbs, and spices. Add more water, if necessary. Follow the instructions for the mode of cooking you choose.

On the stovetop on medium heat, bring the water to a simmer and reduce the heat to low. Cover and let simmer for at least 4 hours and up to 8. Add water as needed so the bones are always covered.

In a slow cooker, set to low, cover, and let cook for 8 hours.

In a pressure cooker or Instant Pot, using your cooker's instructions, bring up to full pressure. Reduce the heat to low, maintaining full pressure, and cook for 2 hours. Allow the pressure to naturally release.

When the broth is done, remove all the bones and the meat and pour the broth through a fine-mesh strainer into a large bowl. Discard the solids and reserve the meat for another use. (You can also refrigerate or freeze the bones and reuse them to make more broth.)

Let the broth cool completely before covering and placing into the refrigerator. When chilled the broth should be very gelatinous.

The broth will keep for 5 days in the refrigerator and 3 or more months in the freezer.

Turkey Bone Broth

Prep time: 15 min. • Cook time: 2 to 8 hours depending on cooking mode • Yield: 1 gallon of broth

3 or more pounds raw or cooked turkey bones or carcasses

2 or more pounds turkey thighs, legs, and/or wings

6 to 8 chicken feet (optional; they'll add a great deal of collagen to your broth)

1/4 cup apple cider vinegar

Purified water

2 to 4 carrots, scrubbed and roughly chopped

3 to 4 celery stalks, including leafy part, roughly chopped

1 medium onion, cut into large chunks

1 to 2 garlic cloves

1 teaspoon dried sage

2 teaspoons Celtic or pink Himalayan salt

1 teaspoon peppercorns

Fat-burning spices you can add for more fat-burning power:

1-inch piece fresh ginger, sliced

Handful of parsley or cilantro

1 teaspoon fresh or ground turmeric

1/16 to 1/8 teaspoon cayenne

1 to 2 teaspoons cumin

Place all the bones into a large stockpot, slow cooker, or pressure cooker. Add the vinegar and enough purified water to cover everything by 1 inch. Add all the vegetables, herbs, and spices. Add more water, if necessary. Follow the instructions for the mode of cooking you choose.

On the stovetop on medium heat, bring the water to a simmer and reduce the heat to low. Cover and let simmer for at least 4 hours and up to 8. Add water as needed so the bones are always covered.

In a slow cooker, set to low, cover, and let cook for 8 hours.

In a pressure cooker or Instant Pot, using your cooker's instructions, bring up to full pressure. Reduce the heat to low, maintaining full pressure, and cook for 2 hours. Allow the pressure to naturally release.

When the broth is done, remove all the bones and the meat and pour the broth through a fine-mesh strainer into a large bowl. Discard the solids and reserve the meat for another use. (You can also refrigerate or freeze the bones and reuse them to make more broth.)

Let the broth cool completely before covering and placing into the refrigerator. When chilled the broth should be very gelatinous.

The broth will keep for 5 days in the refrigerator and 3 or more months in the freezer.

Seafood Bone Broth

Prep time: 15 min. • Cook time: 45 to 65 min. • Yield: 1 gallon of broth

2 tablespoons ghee (see page 57) or pasture-raised butter

2 to 4 carrots, scrubbed and roughly chopped

3 to 4 celery stalks, including leafy part, roughly chopped

1 medium onion, cut into large chunks

2 or more pounds fish carcasses or heads from large nonoily fish (halibut, cod, sole, rockfish, turbot, tilapia, etc.), washed, rinsed, and gills removed

12 or more shrimp shells and tails, washed and rinsed

Purified water

1 tablespoon pickling spice mix

1 teaspoon peppercorns

(recipe continues)

Fat-burning spices you can add for more fat-burning power:

1-inch piece fresh ginger, sliced   **1 teaspoon fresh or ground turmeric**
Handful of parsley or cilantro   **1/16 to 1/8 teaspoon cayenne**

In a large stockpot, melt the ghee over medium-low to low heat. Add the carrots, celery, and onion and cook, stirring occasionally, for about 20 minutes.

Add the fish carcasses and shrimp shells and enough purified water to cover everything by 1 inch. Add the pickling spice and peppercorns and increase the heat to medium. Bring the water to a bare simmer and reduce the heat to low. Use a shallow spoon to skim the film off the top of the broth. Cook for 25 to 40 minutes at a low simmer with the lid askew or uncovered. Continue to skim the surface as needed.

When the broth is done, remove all the bones and shells and pour the broth through a fine-mesh strainer into a large bowl. Discard the solids and let the broth cool completely before covering and placing into the refrigerator. When chilled the broth should be very gelatinous.

The broth will keep for 3 days in the refrigerator and 3 or more months in the freezer.

Note

Because fish bones are so soft and the cooking process so fast, you should not prepare seafood bone broth in a slow cooker or pressure cooker.

Vegetable Broth (for Vegetarian Option)

Prep time: 20 min. • Cook time: 4 to 5 hours • Yield: ½ gallon of broth

7 or 8 celery stalks, cut into 2-inch pieces

4 sweet onions, cut into wedges

4 or 5 large carrots, cut into 2-inch pieces

2 large or 3 medium tomatoes, quartered

1 red bell pepper, seeded and cut into thick slices

3 medium turnips, cut into wedges (optional)

¼ cup olive oil

3 garlic cloves

2 whole cloves

1 bay leaf

5 to 6 peppercorns

1 gallon purified water

Preheat the oven to 425°F. Put the celery, onions, carrots, tomatoes, bell pepper, and turnips (if using) in a large bowl. Pour in the olive oil and toss to coat evenly. Spread the vegetables out in a single layer on 2 or more sheet pans. (When vegetables are packed too closely together they will steam instead of roast, and you'll lose the lovely aromatics released in dry cooking.) Roast for 45 to 60 minutes, turning every 20 minutes. The vegetables should be brown and toasted on the outside and tender on the inside, and the onions should be partially caramelized.

Place the roasted vegetables, garlic, cloves, bay leaf, and peppercorns in a large stock pot and add the purified water.

Bring to a boil and immediately reduce the heat to low and simmer, uncovered, for 3 to 4 hours, or until the broth is reduced by half.

Pour the broth through a fine-mesh strainer into a large bowl. Save the vegetables in a covered container and let the broth cool completely before covering and placing into the refrigerator.

The broth will keep for up to 5 days in the refrigerator and up to 6 months in the freezer.

(recipe continues)

Notes

Roasting fresh vegetables brings out a greatly enhanced flavor profile because of aromatics created while dry roasting, so we roast the vegetables for this broth. It takes a bit more time, but it is so worth that one extra hour in the oven.

The turnips are suggested because they add a bit of spice and a deep earthy flavor.

Save the vegetables from the broth for later use. They're delicious hot or cold!

Broth Variations

You can spice up any of the broth recipes with any of the fat-burning herbs and spices listed on pages 61 and 62 or any variation of the seasonings to create flavors you enjoy.

For a Chinese-style broth try a 2-inch piece of fresh ginger (sliced), scallions, lemongrass, cilantro, Chinese five-spice powder, and white pepper.

To add Thai seasonings try a 2-inch piece of fresh ginger (sliced), lemongrass, scallions, kaffir lime leaves, galangal, and white pepper.

For a spicy broth with Mexican flavors add cilantro, cumin, cayenne, cinnamon, coriander, and jalapeños or other chile peppers.

For an Italian-style broth add tomatoes, Italian seasoning, basil, parsley, marjoram, fennel, anise seed, and oregano.

Broth Loading

Borscht (Russian Cabbage and Beet Soup)

This traditional Eastern European soup combines sweet and sour flavors. The beets offer sweetness and the red wine vinegar adds a bit of tang. Borscht can be served hot or chilled, making it a great all-weather soup. Borscht is one of those love-it-or-hate-it soups. It reminds me of pickled beets and cabbage, so if those flavors are on your list of favorites, you will likely enjoy this soup.

Prep time: 20 min. • Cook time: 40 min. • Yield: 4 servings

2 tablespoons ghee (see page 57) or pasture-raised butter

1 garlic clove, minced

1 medium onion, diced

1 leek, white and pale green parts only, thinly sliced

2 carrots, thinly sliced

2 celery stalks, thinly sliced

¼ to ½ head savoy or green cabbage (about 3 cups)

4 cups Beef Bone Broth (page 178) or Dr. Kellyann's Collagen Broth

1 bay leaf

½ teaspoon dried marjoram

2 medium beets, peeled and grated

1 tablespoon red wine or balsamic vinegar (optional for a sweeter taste)

2 or more tablespoons fresh dill, minced

1½ teaspoons Celtic or pink Himalayan salt

½ teaspoon freshly ground black pepper

In a large stock pot, melt the ghee over medium heat. Add the garlic, onion, and leek and reduce the heat to medium-low. Sauté for about 5 minutes. Add the carrots, celery, and cabbage, raise the heat to medium, and cover, stirring occasionally, for about 10 minutes, until softened.

(recipe continues)

Add the bone broth, bay leaf, and marjoram and simmer for about 10 minutes. Add the beets. Reduce the heat to medium-low and simmer for about 15 minutes, until all the vegetables are tender. Stir in the vinegar, dill, salt, and pepper and serve.

Note
If you like the flavor of caraway seeds (think seeded rye bread), add 1 or 2 teaspoons when you add the carrots, celery, and cabbage.

Butternut Squash Soup

This golden soup takes winter squash to a whole new level. If you don't want to peel and cut up a whole squash, many stores offer the convenience of squash already cubed and ready to cook, saving you time in the kitchen. You can also use kabocha squash, sometimes called Japanese pumpkin because it looks like a stocky green striped pumpkin; it tastes much like a sweet potato.

Prep time: 20 min. • Cook time: 25 min. • Yield: 4 servings

1 tablespoon ghee (see page 57) or pasture-raised butter

1 garlic clove, minced

1 medium onion, diced

1 medium (3-pound) butternut or kabocha squash, cubed (about 4 cups)

2 carrots, sliced

4 cups Chicken (page 179) or Turkey (page 182) Bone Broth or Dr. Kellyann's Collagen Broth

1 sprig fresh sage, or 1/4 teaspoon dried sage

1 teaspoon ground cinnamon

1 teaspoon ground nutmeg

1/8 teaspoon cayenne pepper

2 whole cloves

1-inch piece fresh ginger, peeled and grated

1 (13 1/2- to 15-ounce) can unsweetened full-fat coconut milk

1 teaspoon Celtic or pink Himalayan salt

1/2 teaspoon freshly ground black pepper

In a large stockpot, melt the ghee over medium heat. Add the garlic and onion and sauté for about 5 minutes. Add the squash, carrots, bone broth, sage, cinnamon, nutmeg, cayenne pepper, cloves, and ginger. Bring to a simmer and stir, then reduce the heat to medium-low. Cover, stirring occasionally, for about 20 minutes, until the squash is tender.

Purée with an immersion blender, blender, or food processor until smooth. Return to the stockpot, stir in the coconut milk, and simmer for about 5 minutes, or until warmed through. Add the salt and pepper and taste to adjust the seasoning. Serve warm.

Notes

Use caution when blending hot liquids. If you use a blender or food processor, work in small batches, covering the top of the sealed blender or processor with a clean kitchen towel to avoid getting burned.

This soup is good right after you make it and amazing the next day because the flavors have had time to meld.

Chicken and "Rice" Soup

How can you not like chicken-and-rice soup? It's an all-American staple. It reminds me of when I was a kid and my mom always had a pot of chicken stock around, both for soup and for use in cooking. She would make rice especially for me since I always liked it better than noodles. If you're a noodle lover, swap out the cauliflower for zoodles but don't add them until the very end just to warm them through.

Prep time: 20 min. • Cook time: 25 min. • Yield: 4 servings

2 tablespoons ghee (see page 57) or pasture-raised butter

1 small onion, measured after dicing

1 medium head cauliflower, chopped or pulsed in a food processor into rice-size pieces (4 to 5 cups)

2 celery stalks, diced

2 medium carrots, diced

4 cups Chicken Bone Broth (page 179) or Dr. Kellyann's Collagen Broth

1 (13½- to 15-ounce) can unsweetened full-fat coconut milk

¼ cup fresh parsley, coarsely chopped

1 teaspoon fresh thyme leaves, or about ½ teaspoon dried thyme

1½ teaspoons Celtic or pink Himalayan salt

½ teaspoon freshly ground black pepper

In a large stockpot, melt the ghee over medium-high heat. Add the onion and reduce the heat to medium-low. Sauté for 3 to 5 minutes, until the onions are translucent. Add the cauliflower, celery, and carrots and cook for about 8 minutes, until the vegetables are tender. Add the bone broth, coconut milk, parsley, and thyme and bring to a boil. Immediately reduce the heat to low and simmer for 8 to 10 minutes to warm through. Add the salt and pepper and adjust seasonings to taste. Serve immediately.

Creamy Asparagus Soup

Asparagus offers some serious health perks. It helps promote overall digestive health, a benefit of all that soluble and insoluble fiber. It's also a natural diuretic and helps flush excess liquid from your body. Asparagus is loaded with folic acid, vitamins, and minerals, too.

Prep time: 15 min. • Cook time: 25 min. • Yield: 4 to 6 servings

2 tablespoons ghee (see page 57) or pasture-raised butter

1 garlic clove, minced

2 leeks, white and pale green parts only, thinly sliced

1 celery stalk, sliced

4 cups Chicken Bone Broth (page 179) or Dr. Kellyann's Collagen Broth

1 pound asparagus, cut into 1-inch pieces

1 (13½- to 15-ounce) can unsweetened full-fat coconut milk

Pinch of ground nutmeg, plus more for serving

1 teaspoon Celtic or pink Himalayan salt

½ teaspoon freshly ground black pepper, plus more for serving

1 teaspoon arrowroot, blended with 1 tablespoon water

In a large stockpot, melt the ghee over medium-high heat. Add the garlic, leeks, and celery and reduce the heat to medium-low. Sauté for 6 to 8 minutes to soften. Raise the heat to medium-high and add the bone broth and asparagus. When the soup begins to simmer, reduce the heat to medium-low and simmer for 15 to 20 minutes, until asparagus is tender.

Purée with an immersion blender, blender, or food processor until smooth. Return to the stockpot and stir in the coconut milk, nutmeg, salt, pepper, and arrowroot mixture. Simmer for 3 to 5 minutes, until the soup thickens, adding more arrowroot if a thicker soup is desired. Serve warm and garnish with additional freshly ground black pepper and nutmeg, if desired.

(recipe continues)

Note

Use caution when blending hot liquids. If you use a blender or food processor, work in small batches, covering the top of the sealed blender or food processor with a clean kitchen towel to avoid getting burned.

Creamy Pumpkin Soup with Indian Spices

When autumn shows her glorious colors we think of all things pumpkin, and this soup is no exception. It's a hearty, warming, and aromatic soup perfect for the cooler days. It's also fabulous the next day because the spices have had time to meld and mingle, enhancing the flavors even more.

Prep time: 20 min. • Cook time: 25 min. • Yield: 4 servings

1 tablespoon coconut oil, ghee (see page 57), or pasture-raised butter

1 medium onion, diced (about 1½ cups), measured after dicing

2 garlic cloves, minced

2 celery stalks, rough chopped

1-inch piece fresh ginger, peeled and minced (about 2 teaspoons; not dried powdered ginger)

2 teaspoons ground cumin

1 teaspoon ground coriander

⅛ teaspoon ground cardamom

½ teaspoon red pepper flakes

2 (15-ounce) cans pumpkin (not pie filling), or about 4 cups roasted pumpkin

4 cups Chicken Bone Broth (page 179) or Dr. Kellyann's Collagen Broth

1 (13½- to 15-ounce) can unsweetened full-fat coconut milk

1½ teaspoons Celtic or pink Himalayan salt

2 tablespoons toasted pumpkin seeds, for garnish (optional)

In a large stockpot, melt the coconut oil over medium heat. Add the onion, garlic, and celery and sauté for 3 to 5 minutes, until the onions are translucent. Add the ginger, cumin, coriander, cardamom, and red pepper flakes and cook for about 5 minutes, or until the spices are fragrant.

Add the pumpkin and bone broth and bring to a simmer. Reduce the heat to low and let simmer for 15 to 20 minutes.

Purée with an immersion blender, blender, or food processor until smooth. Return to the stockpot, stir in the coconut milk, and warm through. Add salt and pepper and taste to adjust the seasoning. Serve immediately. Garnish with a few toasted pumpkin seeds (if using).

Notes

A fresh 3-pound pie pumpkin will yield about 2 cups of pumpkin purée.

Use caution when blending hot liquids. If you use a blender or food processor, process in small batches, covering the top of the blender or food processor with a clean kitchen towel to avoid getting burned.

This soup is even better on the second day after the spices have had time to mingle.

Roasted Curried Cauliflower Soup

Curry powder is a combination of aromatic spices, not just one spice. There are a variety of combinations, but they often contain coriander, cumin, turmeric, fenugreek, and chile peppers. There's a vast array of other spices that are sometimes used in curry: ginger, caraway, garlic, cinnamon, nutmeg, curry leaf, and black pepper. Curries always combine warming spices, which have a number of health benefits.

Prep time: 20 min. • Cook time: 45 min. • Yield: 4 to 6 servings

1 medium head cauliflower, cut into florets

1/2 medium onion, quartered and separated

2 garlic cloves, minced

1/4 cup olive oil

2 tablespoons red wine vinegar

1 tablespoon curry powder

1/2 tablespoon paprika

1 teaspoon Celtic or pink Himalayan salt

1/2 teaspoon freshly ground black pepper

1/4 teaspoon fresh or ground turmeric

4 cups Chicken Bone Broth (page 179) or Dr. Kellyann's Collagen Broth

1/2 cup canned unsweetened full-fat coconut milk

1/8 cup cilantro, chopped (optional)

Preheat the oven to 400°F. In a large bowl, place the cauliflower, onion, and garlic. In a small bowl, combine the oil, vinegar, curry powder, paprika, salt, pepper, and turmeric and whisk until well blended. Pour the oil mixture over the cauliflower mixture. Toss to coat evenly and spread out in one layer on two sheet pans, leaving plenty of room around the vegetables. Roast for about 40 minutes, turning once halfway through. The vegetables should be brown and toasted on the outside and tender on the inside.

In a large stockpot, combine the roasted vegetables and bone broth. Purée with an immersion blender, blender, or food processor until smooth. Return to the stockpot, stir in the coconut milk, and warm through. Garnish with the cilantro (if using) and serve immediately.

Notes

When roasting the vegetables be sure not to pack them too close together, as they will steam instead of roast, and you'll lose the lovely aromatics released in dry cooking.

Use caution when blending hot liquids. If you use a blender or food processor, process in small batches, covering the top of the blender or food processor with a clean kitchen towel to avoid getting burned.

The flavors bloom overnight so this soup will taste even better on the second day.

Detox Veggie Soup

All these good-for-you vegetables, coupled with ginger, turmeric, cinnamon, and cayenne pepper, will keep your metabolism revved up and help the pounds melt off. You can add or subtract vegetables based on your personal preferences as long as the veggies are on the approved vegetable list. Bon appétit!

Prep time: 20 min. • Cook time: 35 min. • Yield: 6 servings

2 tablespoons olive oil, plus more for serving

1 garlic clove, minced

1 medium onion, diced

6 cups Chicken Bone Broth (page 179) or Dr. Kellyann's Collagen Broth

2 carrots, thinly sliced

2 celery stalks, thinly sliced

1 cup broccoli or cauliflower florets, cut into ½-inch pieces

1 cup kale, stems removed, cut into ribbons

1 cup cabbage, cut into ribbons

8 cherry tomatoes, halved

½ cup parsley or basil, roughly chopped

1-inch piece fresh ginger, peeled and grated

1 teaspoon fresh or ground turmeric

½ teaspoon ground cinnamon

Pinch or more of cayenne pepper

2 teaspoons Celtic or pink Himalayan salt

1 teaspoon freshly ground black pepper

(recipe continues)

In a large stockpot, warm the olive oil over medium-high heat. Add the garlic and onion and sauté for 3 to 5 minutes, until the onion is translucent. Add the bone broth, carrots, celery, broccoli, kale, cabbage, tomatoes, parsley, ginger, turmeric, cinnamon, cayenne pepper, salt, and black pepper and bring to a simmer. Reduce the heat to low and cover, stirring occasionally, for 20 to 30 minutes, until the vegetables are tender. Ladle the soup into a bowl and drizzle with 1 teaspoon of the olive oil.

Lemony Chicken Vegetable

Lemon offers so many health benefits—it promotes hydration and weight loss, provides lots of vitamin C, and aids digestion, to name just a few. Coupled with all the benefits of bone broth and a healthy serving of vegetables, this soup is sure to please. I call this my feel-good soup.

Prep time: 20 min. • Cook time: 25 min. • Yield: 4 to 6 servings

2 tablespoons ghee (see page 57) or pasture-raised butter

1 garlic clove, minced

1 leek, white and pale green parts only, thinly sliced

4 cups Chicken Bone Broth (page 179) or Dr. Kellyann's Collagen Broth

2 carrots, sliced

2 celery stalks, sliced

1 to 2 cups zucchini and/or yellow summer squash, diced

2 teaspoons lemon zest

2 tablespoons fresh lemon juice

¼ cup parsley or basil, coarsely chopped

1 teaspoon herbes de Provence

1 teaspoon Celtic or pink Himalayan salt

½ teaspoon freshly ground black pepper

2 cups or more loosely packed baby spinach

Lemon wedges, for serving

In a large stockpot, melt the ghee over medium-high heat. Add the garlic and leeks and sauté for 3 to 5 minutes on medium heat. Add the bone broth, carrots, celery, zucchini, lemon zest, lemon juice, parsley, herbes de Provence, salt, and pepper and bring to a simmer. Reduce the heat to low and cover, stirring occasionally, for about 20 minutes, or until the carrots are tender. Stir in the spinach and serve with lemon wedges.

Roasted Vegetable Soup

Roasting or dry-heat cooking helps release the natural sugars in vegetables. This caramelization happens when there is no water used in cooking. The sugars in the vegetables break down from the heat, creating hundreds of aromatic compounds that produce a range of complex flavors. Roasting vegetables before adding them to your bone broth adds all those deep, rich flavors to the soup.

Prep time: 20 min. • Cook time: 40 min. • Yield: 4 to 6 servings

2 cups butternut or kabocha squash, cut into ½-inch pieces

1 cup broccoli florets, cut into ½-inch pieces

1 to 2 zucchini, halved lengthwise and sliced into thick quarter- to half-inch half-moons (about 1 cup)

1 cup cauliflower florets, cut into ½-inch pieces

1 medium sweet onion, sliced ½-inch thick

¼ cup olive oil

1 teaspoon or more bouquet garni, herbes de Provence, or Italian seasoning

1½ teaspoon Celtic or pink Himalayan salt

½ teaspoon freshly ground black pepper

4 cups Chicken (page 179), Turkey (page 182), or Beef (page 178) Bone Broth or Dr. Kellyann's Collagen Broth

Preheat the oven to 425°F. In a large bowl, place the squash, broccoli, zucchini, cauliflower, and onion and then pour in the olive oil, seasonings, salt, and pepper. Toss to coat evenly and spread out in one

(recipe continues)

layer on two sheet pans, leaving plenty of room around the vegetables. Roast the vegetables for 30 to 40 minutes, turning once halfway through. They should be brown and toasted on the outside and tender on the inside.

In a large stockpot, pour the bone broth and place over medium-high heat. When the broth begins to simmer, add the vegetables, reduce the heat, and bring back to a simmer. Taste and adjust the seasoning to your liking. Serve immediately.

Notes

Because different vegetables take different times to roast, be sure you cut the butternut or kabocha squash into very small pieces to shorten their roasting time. That's the same reason the zucchini is cut into thicker pieces. Basically the harder the vegetable, the longer its roasting time.

When roasting the vegetables be sure not to pack them too close together, as they will steam instead of roast, and you'll lose the lovely aromatics released in dry cooking.

You can also keep the roasted vegetables in the refrigerator until you're ready for a bowl of soup. Spoon out enough vegetables to fill your soup bowl half full, ladle in bone broth, and warm on the stovetop to heat through, making one serving at a time.

You can also add or substitute any of your favorite non-starchy vegetables.

Depending on how many vegetables you use, you may want to add more bone broth.

Thai Red Curry Soup

Hearty, healthy, and velvety smooth, Thai Red Curry Soup is one of my favorite meals when I'm in the mood for something with a bit of spice. When you're cooking with curry, a bit of sweetness can help balance the spice.

Prep time: 15 min. • Cook time: 25 min. • Yield: 4 servings

1 tablespoon coconut oil

2 garlic cloves, smashed

1 small onion, thinly sliced

1 red bell pepper, cut into thin strips

3 baby bok choy, coarsely chopped

3 to 4 ounces white, cremini, and/or shitake mushrooms, sliced (about 1 cup)

1-inch piece fresh ginger, peeled and grated

1 to 1½ tablespoons Thai red curry paste

4 cups Chicken Bone Broth (page 179) or Dr. Kellyann's Collagen Broth

1 (13½- to 15-ounce) can unsweetened full-fat coconut milk

1 tablespoon fish sauce

Stevia or monk fruit sweetener, to equal 2 to 3 teaspoons sugar

3 green onions, white and green parts, thinly sliced

⅓ cup cilantro leaves

¼ cup basil leaves

Juice of ½ lime (about 2 tablespoons)

1 teaspoon Celtic or pink Himalayan salt

½ teaspoon freshly ground white pepper

In a large stockpot, melt the coconut oil over medium heat. Add the garlic, onion, bell pepper, bok choy, and mushrooms and sauté 8 to 10 minutes, until softened. Add the ginger and red curry paste and cook until fragrant, about 1 to 2 minutes. Stir in the bone broth and coconut milk.

Bring to a boil and immediately reduce the heat to low. Simmer for about 10 minutes to meld the flavors. Stir in the fish sauce and sweetener. Remove from the heat and add the green onions, cilantro, basil, lime juice, salt, and white pepper. Taste and adjust the seasonings to your liking. Serve immediately.

(recipe continues)

Notes

A delicious serving suggestion is to pour the soup over warmed cauliflower rice for a heartier soup.

If you haven't cooked much with Thai red curry paste, it's best to start with less, especially if it's very fresh. You can always add more. Start with 1 tablespoon and adjust at the end. The flavors bloom overnight, so the soup is even better on the second day.

You can find Thai red curry paste in the Asian section of most grocery stores. It is usually packaged in a small jar.

This is another great soup you can make as an entrée after you complete the cleanse. Simply add peeled and deveined shrimp or chicken, about 3 to 4 ounces per person. Right after you melt the coconut oil in the first step, sauté thinly sliced raw chicken or shrimp for about 3 minutes. Then continue with the recipe as written. If you are adding rotisserie chicken or fully cooked chicken or shrimp, add it to the stockpot when you add the broth.

Tom Kha Gai (Chicken Coconut Soup)

You know that wonderful creamy soup served in Thai restaurants that comes to the table simmering in a pot heated with a flame? This is it! It is traditionally served tableside to two or more people, creating a perfect community meal. Now you can serve it at home, and it's so easy to make.

Prep time: 15 min. • Cook time: 25 min. • Yield: 4 servings

1 tablespoon coconut oil

1 lemongrass stalk, cut into 2-inch pieces

1-inch piece fresh ginger, peeled and thinly sliced

8 kaffir lime leaves, or 1 tablespoon lime zest plus 2 tablespoons fresh lime juice

1 celery stalk, sliced

4 cups Chicken Bone Broth (page 179) or Dr. Kellyann's Collagen Broth

8 to 12 ounces white, cremini, shiitake, oyster, and/or maitake mushrooms, sliced (about 3 to 4 cups)

1 (13½- to 15-ounce) can unsweetened full-fat coconut milk

1½ tablespoons fish sauce

½ teaspoon Celtic or pink Himalayan salt

⅛ teaspoon crushed red pepper flakes, plus more for garnish

½ teaspoon freshly ground white pepper

¼ cup cilantro, coarsely chopped, plus more for garnish

Stevia or monk fruit sweetener, to equal 1 teaspoon sugar

Fresh lime wedges

In a large stockpot, melt the coconut oil over medium-high heat. Add the lemongrass, ginger, kaffir leaves, celery, and bone broth. Bring to a boil and reduce the heat to low. Simmer for about 10 minutes to meld the flavors. Strain the broth into a large bowl and discard the solids.

Return the broth to the stockpot and add the mushrooms. Simmer for another 5 minutes until the mushrooms are tender. Stir in the coconut milk, fish sauce, salt, red pepper flakes, pepper, cilantro, and sweetener and warm through. Taste and adjust the seasonings to your liking. Garnish with the crushed red pepper flakes, cilantro, and fresh lime wedges.

(recipe continues)

Notes

Green vegetables are not traditionally used in this soup, but you can add 1 to 2 cups broccoli florets, 2 to 3 cups roughly chopped baby bok choy, or 2 to 3 cups baby spinach. Add the greens when you add the mushrooms.

This is a great soup to turn into an entrée after you're done with the cleanse. Simply add very thinly sliced pieces of raw or precooked chicken breast (about 4 ounces per person) when you add the broth to the stockpot. If you use raw chicken, simmer the broth for 8 to 10 minutes to fully cook the chicken. You can also use shredded or thinly sliced rotisserie chicken.

Creamy Tomato Florentine Soup

Prep time: 15 min. • Cook time: 25 min. • Yield: 4 to 6 servings

4 cups Chicken Bone Broth (page 179) or Dr. Kellyann's Collagen Broth

1 (28-ounce) can diced tomatoes

1 garlic clove, smashed

½ cup canned unsweetened full-fat coconut milk

2 teaspoons Italian seasoning

3 cups or more loosely packed baby spinach

1 cup fresh basil leaves, cut into fine ribbons

1 teaspoon Celtic or pink Himalayan salt

½ teaspoon freshly ground black pepper

In a large stockpot, heat the bone broth over medium-high heat. Pour the canned tomatoes into a blender and purée until smooth. Add the tomatoes and garlic to the broth and bring to a simmer. Add the coconut milk and Italian seasoning and reduce the heat to low. Simmer for 15 to 20 minutes. Add the spinach, basil, salt, and pepper and simmer for another 3 minutes. Serve warm.

Chilled Cucumber Soup

Prep time: 15 min. • Cook time: 12 min. • Yield: 4 to 6 servings

1 cup water

4 medium cucumbers, peeled, seeded, and sliced

1/2 cup sliced yellow onion

1 teaspoon Celtic or pink Himalayan salt

1/2 teaspoon freshly ground black pepper

4 cups Chicken Bone Broth (page 179) or Dr. Kellyann's Collagen Broth

1/2 teaspoon arrowroot powder, blended with 1 teaspoon water

1 small bay leaf

1 cup unsweetened plain almond milk

1 teaspoon minced fresh dill

1 teaspoon minced fresh Italian parsley

1 teaspoon minced fresh chives

1/2 teaspoon fresh lemon zest

In a large stockpot, bring the water to a boil over medium-high heat. Add the cucumbers, onion, salt, and pepper and cover. Simmer for 5 to 7 minutes, until the vegetables are very soft.

Purée using a food processor, blender, or immersion blender until smooth. In a large stockpot, bring the bone broth to a simmer and add the arrowroot mixture, bay leaf, and puréed cucumbers. Reduce the heat to low and simmer, stirring for 5 minutes, until the soup thickens. Let the soup cool to room temperature and add the almond milk, fresh herbs, and lemon zest. Refrigerate. Serve the soup very cold.

Note

Use caution when puréeing hot soup in a blender or food processor. Work in small batches and cover the top of the sealed blender or processor with a kitchen towel to avoid getting burned.

Creamy Broccoli Soup

Prep time: 15 min. • Cook time: 25 min. • Yield: 4 to 6 servings

2 tablespoons ghee (see page 57) or pasture-raised butter

2 cloves garlic, minced

1 small onion, diced

4 cups Chicken Bone Broth (page 179) or Dr. Kellyann's Collagen Broth

1 cup canned unsweetened full-fat coconut milk

4 cups broccoli florets

½ teaspoon ground nutmeg

1 teaspoon Celtic or pink Himalayan salt

½ teaspoon freshly ground black pepper

In a large stockpot, melt the ghee over medium-high heat. Add the garlic and onion and reduce the heat to medium-low. Cook, stirring, for 6 to 8 minutes, until softened.

Raise the heat to medium-high and add the bone broth, coconut milk, broccoli, nutmeg, salt, and pepper. When the soup begins to simmer, reduce the heat to medium-low and simmer for 15 to 20 minutes, until the broccoli is cooked through.

Purée with a hand-held immersion blender, blender, or food processor until smooth and creamy. Serve warm.

Note

Use caution when puréeing soup in a blender or food processor. Work in small batches and cover the top of the sealed blender or processor with a kitchen towel to avoid getting burned.

Watercress Soup

Prep time: 10 min. • Cook time: 10 min. • Yield: 4 to 6 servings

2 tablespoons ghee (see page 57)
or pasture-raised butter

1 medium onion, diced

2 garlic cloves, minced

4 cups Chicken Bone Broth
(page 179) or Dr. Kellyann's
Collagen Broth

1/2 to 1 teaspoon Celtic or
pink Himalayan salt

1/2 teaspoon freshly ground
black or white pepper

1/2 cup canned unsweetened
full-fat coconut milk (optional,
for a creamier soup)

2 bunches of watercress (about
14 ounces), thick stems removed

In a large stockpot, melt the ghee over medium-high heat. Add the onion and garlic, reduce the heat to medium-low, and cook, stirring, for 6 to 8 minutes, until softened.

Raise the heat to medium-high and add the bone broth, salt, and pepper. If using the coconut milk, add it now. Bring to a boil, then reduce the heat to medium low and simmer for 3 minutes. Add the watercress and simmer for about 1 minute, just to wilt the watercress. Watercress soup can be served as is or puréed. Purée with an immersion blender, blender, or food processor until smooth and creamy.

Note

Use caution when puréeing soup in a blender or food processor. Work in small batches and cover the top of the sealed blender or processor with a kitchen towel to avoid getting burned.

Cauliflower Vichyssoise

Prep time: 15 min. • Cook time: 25 min. • Yield: 4 to 6 servings

2 tablespoons ghee (see page 57) or pasture-raised butter

1 garlic clove, minced

2 leeks, white and pale green parts only, thinly sliced

4 cups Chicken Bone Broth (page 179) or Dr. Kellyann's Collagen Broth

1/2 cup canned unsweetened full-fat coconut milk

3 cups cauliflower florets

1/2 teaspoon dried thyme

1 teaspoon Celtic or pink Himalayan salt

1/2 teaspoon freshly ground black pepper, plus more for serving

1/2 teaspoon arrowroot powder, blended with 1 tablespoon water, plus more if needed

In a large stockpot, melt the ghee over medium-high heat. Add the garlic and leeks and reduce the heat to medium-low. Cook, stirring, for 6 to 8 minutes, until softened.

Raise the heat to medium-high and add the bone broth, coconut milk, cauliflower, thyme, salt, and pepper. When the soup begins to simmer, reduce the heat to medium-low and simmer for 15 to 20 minutes, until the cauliflower is cooked through.

Purée with an immersion blender, blender, or food processor until smooth and creamy. Return to the stockpot and stir in the arrowroot mixture. Simmer for 3 to 5 minutes, until the soup thickens, adding more arrowroot if a thicker soup is desired. Serve warm, garnished with freshly ground black pepper.

Note

Use caution when puréeing soup in a blender or food processor. Work in small batches and cover the top of the sealed blender or processor with a kitchen towel to avoid getting burned.

Chapter 10

Refreshing Detox Waters

Healing foods are a big key to your cleanse, but you know what's just as important? Hydration, hydration, hydration! I want you to load up on water every day, and here's why.

In your bloodstream, water carries nutrients and oxygen to your cells. In your digestive system, it helps you digest food and flushes out toxins. Water lubricates your joints and acts as a "shock absorber" for your tissues, and it keeps your skin moist and supple.

What's more, drinking water can help you lose weight. One study found that drinking about two cups of water increases your metabolic rate by up to 30% and keeps it elevated for an hour.[1] Drinking water also fills you up, so you can eat less and still feel satisfied—an effect you can't get from drinking diet sodas. One group of researchers found that women who drank a glass of water after lunch each day while they were dieting lost significantly more weight than women who drank diet beverages with their meals.[2]

Unfortunately, water gets short shrift in our diets these days, with research suggesting that up to 75% of us are chronically dehydrated.[3] Chronic dehydration causes "brain fog" and a host of other problems ranging from headaches to constipation to muscle cramps. In addition, it dries out your skin and makes your eyes look sunken, adding years to your age.

Luckily, dehydration is one of the easiest problems to solve. On your cleanse, you'll get lots of water from your broth and morning lemon water. In addition, I want you to drink about half your body weight in ounces of water each day, plus more if you've been sweating while exercising or doing yard work. This is especially important because a low-carb diet has diuretic effects.

You can drink your water "straight" or in coffee or tea—or, for bonus cleansing points, you can make beautiful detox waters infused with the flavors of fresh fruit, veggies, and herbs. If you're not familiar with detox water, it's any infused water (i.e., water flavored by submerging fruit, vegetables, herbs, and spices in it) that helps flush your system of toxins and improves your health. The added ingredients can add a nutritional boost—for instance, revving up your metabolism—but the main beneficial ingredient is water.

There's no end to the flavor combinations you can create when you make detox water. So in addition to trying my recipes, invent your own; it's a great way to use up odds and ends from your fruit bowl and vegetable bin. Here is a list of combinations you may want to try:

- Cantaloupe and strawberry
- Cucumber and mint
- Fresh lavender and lemon
- Green tea and ginger
- Green tea, lemon, and ginger
- Lemon and ginger
- Lemon and lime
- Lemon and raspberry
- Lemon and thyme
- Lemon, lime, and grapefruit
- Lemon, lime, or orange and mint
- Lime, cilantro, and cayenne

- Mixed berries
- Orange and blueberry
- Orange and fennel
- Orange and raspberry
- Peach and thyme
- Peach, plum, and nectarine
- Pineapple and mango
- Strawberry and peach
- Watermelon and mint

You can use a pitcher to make your detox water, following the instructions in the recipes, or you can use an infuser bottle. If you use an infuser bottle, just reduce your ingredients accordingly. Either way, you're going to love these sparkly, fresh drinks—and your cells will love all the water you're sending their way!

Oh, and here's a tip: once you're on Dr. Kellyann's Lifestyle Plan, you can add a dose of collagen to your detox water. It's an easy way to get your daily collagen fix.

Apple Cinnamon Detox Water

Prep time: 5 min. • Yield: 8 servings

1 apple, cored and thinly sliced

1 cinnamon stick

3 cups or more of ice, enough to fill a pitcher halfway

Enough purified water to fill a 2-quart (½ gallon) pitcher

Place the apple and cinnamon stick in a pitcher and top with the ice (this will keep the fruit submerged). Fill the pitcher with the purified water. Refrigerate for at least 2 hours so the flavors can meld. The flavors will continue to develop over time. As you drink the detox water,

(recipe continues)

you can continue to add water to the pitcher until the fruit no longer infuses the water with flavor.

Note

Use a cinnamon stick instead of ground cinnamon, which won't fully dissolve.

Grapefruit and Rosemary Detox Water

Prep time: 5 min. • Yield: 8 servings

1/2 unpeeled grapefruit, sliced

2 to 4 sprigs rosemary

3 cups or more of ice, enough to fill a pitcher halfway

Enough purified water to fill a 2-quart (1/2 gallon) pitcher

Place the grapefruit and rosemary in a pitcher and top with the ice (this will keep the fruit submerged). Fill the pitcher with the purified water. Refrigerate for at least 2 hours so the flavors can meld. The flavors will continue to develop over time. As you drink the detox water, you can continue to add water to the pitcher until the fruit no longer infuses the water with flavor.

Note

Rosemary also works well with pears. Swap out the grapefruit for 1 thinly sliced pear (my favorites are red pears).

Lemon and Cucumber Detox Water

Prep time: 5 min. • Yield: 8 servings

1 to 2 lemons, sliced

1 medium cucumber, sliced

3 cups or more of ice, enough to fill a pitcher halfway

Enough purified water to fill a 2-quart (1/2 gallon) pitcher

Place the lemon and cucumber in a pitcher and top with the ice (this will keep the fruit submerged). Fill the pitcher with the purified water. Refrigerate for at least 2 hours so the flavors can meld. The flavors will continue to develop over time. As you drink the detox water, you can continue to add water to the pitcher until the fruit no longer infuses the water with flavor.

Notes

To enhance the water you can add a handful of mint leaves or 1/2 teaspoon of ground turmeric.

You can also add a pinch of cayenne pepper if you like spice.

Prefer limes? Use them in place of the lemons.

Pineapple and Strawberry Detox Water

Prep time: 5 min. • Yield: 8 servings

1 cup fresh, frozen, or canned unsweetened pineapple chunks

1 cup fresh or frozen strawberries

3 cups or more of ice, enough to fill a pitcher halfway

Enough purified water to fill a 2-quart (1/2 gallon) pitcher

Place the pineapple and strawberries in the bottom of a pitcher and top with the ice (this will keep the fruit submerged). Fill the pitcher

(recipe continues)

with the purified water. Refrigerate for at least 2 hours so the flavors can meld. The flavors will continue to develop over time. As you drink the detox water, you can continue to add water to the pitcher until the fruit no longer infuses the water with flavor.

Strawberry Lemon Basil Detox Water

Prep time: 5 min. • Yield: 8 servings

1 cup of fresh or frozen strawberries

1/2 lemon, sliced

A small handful of basil, 6 to 8 leaves, scrunched in your hand (to release the aromatic oils)

3 cups or more of ice, enough to fill a pitcher halfway

Enough purified water to fill a 2-quart (1/2 gallon) pitcher

Place the strawberries, lemon, and basil in a pitcher and top with the ice (this will keep the fruit and basil submerged). Fill the pitcher with the purified water. Refrigerate for at least 2 hours so the flavors can meld. The flavors will continue to develop over time. As you drink the detox water, you can continue to add water to the pitcher until the fruit no longer infuses the water with flavor.

Chapter 11

Recipes for Dr. Kellyann's Lifestyle Plan

As soon as you finish your cleanse (and take off any extra pounds with my Bone Broth Diet or 10-Day Belly Slimdown), you're ready to start on Dr. Kellyann's Lifestyle Plan (see Chapter 5). This plan is your secret to staying young, vibrant, and energetic and still getting to enjoy the foods you love. It's how you're going to eat *fearlessly* for life.

Now, a deal's a deal, and earlier I told you that once you're on your maintenance plan, you can eat anything you want for 20% of your meals (as long as you stick to reasonable portions). So yes—you can eat pizza or toaster pancakes or potato chips a couple of times a week. You have my blessing.

However, I'm hoping that even for your 20% meals, you'll frequently skip the junk and opt for foods that your body loves. The more you eat the natural foods that keep your body clean and healthy, the less you'll crave the foods that make it sluggish and sick.

That's why this chapter is all about 20% meals that taste a little bit naughty—from Mocha Collagen Mug Cake (page 219) to Chicken Saltimbocca (page 223)—but still feed your body nutrients it craves. Enjoy!

Apple Cinnamon Mug Cake

Tired of having eggs every morning for breakfast? Here's a sweet treat to change up the morning. This is also a fabulous dessert when you're on a maintenance program.

Prep time: 5 min. • Cook time: 2½ min. • Yield: 1 serving

¼ cup almond flour

¼ cup unsweetened applesauce

1 egg

1 packet Dr. Kellyann's Vanilla Collagen Shake or 1 scoop Dr. Kellyann's Vanilla Bone Broth Protein (or 15 to 25 grams of high-quality vanilla collagen protein powder)

¼ teaspoon ground cinnamon

½ teaspoon baking powder

Coconut oil cooking spray

In a small bowl, combine the flour, applesauce, egg, collagen powder, cinnamon, and baking powder. Spray a large coffee mug with coconut oil. Pour in the batter. Microwave on high for about 2½ minutes. The cake will rise in the mug as it bakes but will deflate when done cooking. Let cool for a few minutes before enjoying. The mug will be extremely hot.

Because grains have so many downsides, it's a smart idea to minimize them in your diet, or even cut them out entirely. But I won't lie: giving up grains is a *big* lifestyle change—and that's especially true if you love baking.

So if you're hesitating to let go of grains entirely, I understand. But the good news is that you can still eat the foods you love! In fact, I think you'll be amazed at what you can make with grain-free flours.

The trick is to stop thinking that *flour equals grains*. There's a whole world of flours and thickeners that don't contain grains, and they're all delicious. Here's an introduction to them.

Almond Flour

Almond flour is made from whole almonds. It's very different from blanched almond flour (see page 216) so make sure you don't confuse the two. Regular almond flour is heavier and more "mealy" than blanched almond flour, so it's best to save it for breading, pie crusts, or cookie recipes that specifically call for it.

Arrowroot Powder

Want to make gravy or thicken soups and sauces without using wheat flour or corn starch? Then this is your answer. However, don't use arrowroot powder with dairy products because it'll turn slimy.

To thicken a sauce with arrowroot, mix it with an equal amount of cold water. Then whisk the mixture into a hot liquid for about half a minute. (Don't mix it directly into hot liquid or it'll clump.) Avoid overheating sauces that contain arrowroot powder because they'll break down and separate.

You can replace flour with arrowroot powder on a one-to-one basis. If you're replacing cornstarch, use a little less.

You can also add arrowroot powder to baked goods containing almond flour or coconut flour. It acts a little like gluten, making them spongier and less crumbly.

Blanched Almond Flour

This flour, made from skinned almonds, is excellent for everything from muffins and quick breads to cookies, brownies, and graham crackers. In addition, you can make a killer pizza crust with it.

The fineness of almond flour's grind varies from brand to brand, and the finest grind will typically give you the best results. To keep your flour fresh, store it in the freezer—but make sure you bring it to room temperature before you bake with it or it'll be "clumpy." You can try substituting it on a one-to-one basis for wheat flour in your recipes, but you'll get much better results with recipes specifically designed for almond flour.

In addition to baking with blanched almond flour, you can bread meats with it. (I use it to bind fritters, too.) Just watch carefully when you brown coated meats because they can burn easily.

Coconut Flour

This is a great go-to flour for waffles, cookies, cakes, and muffins. I also use it to replace bread crumbs in recipes like meatballs and crab cakes. It's so versatile that it should definitely be a staple in any grain-free kitchen.

Coconut flour soaks up liquids like a sponge, so use it in recipes that contain a large amount of wet ingredients. You'll generally need one cup of liquid and several eggs for each cup of coconut flour you use. Sift the flour before you use it to remove any lumps—and let a batter made with coconut flour "rest" a bit before putting it in the oven because it'll thicken up.

Cooking with coconut flour is an art, and tiny changes in your measurements can lead to big changes in your results. So I recommend sticking with simple recipes until you get the hang of it.

Other Nut and Seed Flours

If you want to be adventurous (and you have a little extra cash) try substituting hazelnut or chestnut flour for almond flour. It'll give your baked goods a whole different nutty dimension.

And if you're allergic to nuts, try sunflower seed flour instead. There's just one thing to know ahead of time: sunflower seeds contain chlorogenic acid, and if you mix sunflower seed flour with enough baking soda or baking powder, your baked goods may develop green speckles when they cool. This is totally harmless, but it does look strange!

Plantain Flour and Plantains

Plantain is another fun flour for crepes or pancakes, and some people use it to make tortillas. It has a distinctive taste that most people like. It's not easy to find this flour in stores, but you can order it online.

You can also use puréed green plantains in baking. Plantains aren't bananas—but they look like them, and you'll find them in the banana section of your store's produce department. The greener they are, the better, because they'll taste more neutral and less "banana-ish."

Tapioca Starch

Tapioca starch makes breads containing coconut or almond flour "bouncier" because it adds elasticity. You can also use it on its own to make terrific crepes, pancakes, and flatbreads.

Be Ready for Some Trial and Error

Baking with grain-free flours and thickeners takes practice. You may have a few flops, but pretty soon you'll find that it's just as easy as baking with grain-based flours.

You'll also discover that the Internet is loaded with grain-free baking recipes. (By the way, while you're getting grains out of your life, also look for recipes that replace sugar with healthier sweeteners, such as honey, blackstrap molasses, maple syrup, and fruit.) Before long, you'll be a pro at using your new ingredients—and you'll never miss grain-based flours again.

Latte Collagen Mug Cake

A great breakfast treat when you want something different. You don't have to go to a coffee shop to have a latte. This is also a fabulous dessert when you're on a maintenance plan.

Prep time: 5 min. • Cook time: 2 to 2½ min. • Yield: 1 serving

¼ cup almond flour

½ mashed banana (optional)

1 egg

1 packet Dr. Kellyann's Vanilla Collagen Shake or 1 scoop Dr. Kellyann's Vanilla Bone Broth Protein (or 15 to 25 grams of high-quality vanilla collagen protein powder)

1 teaspoon espresso powder or 1 packet Instant Collagen Coffee

½ teaspoon baking powder

Coconut oil cooking spray

In a small bowl, combine the flour, banana (if using), egg, collagen powder, espresso powder, and baking powder. Spray a large coffee mug with the cooking spray. Pour in the batter. Microwave for about 2½ minutes if using the banana or about 2 minutes without the banana.

The cake will rise as it bakes but will deflate when done cooking. Let cool for a few minutes before enjoying. The mug will be extremely hot.

Mocha Collagen Mug Cake

This mug cake was inspired by my favorite very special coffee drink. What could be better than chocolate and coffee? This is another delicious dessert you can enjoy while on maintenance.

Prep time: 5 min. • Cook time: 2 to 2½ min. • Yield: 1 serving

¼ cup almond flour

½ mashed banana (optional)

1 egg

1 packet Dr. Kellyann's Chocolate Collagen Shake or 1 scoop Dr. Kellyann's Chocolate Bone Broth Protein (or 15 to 25 grams of high-quality chocolate collagen protein powder)

1 teaspoon espresso powder or 1 packet Instant Collagen Coffee

½ teaspoon baking powder

Coconut oil cooking spray

In a small bowl, combine the flour, banana (if using), egg, collagen powder, espresso powder, and baking powder. Spray a large coffee mug with the cooking spray. Pour in the batter. Microwave for about 2½ minutes if using the banana or about 2 minutes without the banana. The cake will rise as it bakes but will deflate when done cooking. Let cool for a few minutes before enjoying. The mug will be extremely hot.

Butternut Breakfast Hash

You know how easy it is to get in a breakfast rut. You make the same thing every morning and eventually you need a change. Try a breakfast hash! You can make a large skillet and divide it up into individual servings to save you time in the morning. It's easy to reheat on the stovetop or in the microwave.

Prep time: 20 min. • Cook time: 30 min. • Yield: 4 servings

4 slices sugar-, nitrate-, and nitrite-free turkey or pork bacon, diced

2 tablespoons olive oil

About 3 pounds butternut or kabocha squash, peeled and diced in ¼-inch pieces (4 cups)

1 red bell pepper, cut into a ¼-inch dice

1 onion, cut into a ¼-inch dice

1 teaspoon Celtic or pink Himalayan salt

½ teaspoon freshly ground black pepper

1 garlic clove, minced (optional)

4 to 6 cups baby spinach

Cook the bacon in a large skillet until crisp. Set the bacon aside on a plate lined with paper towels. In the same skillet, add the olive oil, squash, bell pepper, onion, salt, and pepper and sauté over medium heat for about 8 minutes. Stir in the garlic (if using) and continue cooking for 1 minute more. Add the spinach and bacon, mix well, and sauté for about 1 minute, until spinach begins to wilt.

Notes

Peeling and dicing the squash takes time because it is a very hard vegetable. You can dice it ahead and store in the refrigerator in a sealed bowl filled with water for 1 to 2 days. Drain well before using.

Once prepared, the hash will keep in the refrigerator for 3 to 4 days.

Pumpkin Pecan Pancakes

I can still eat pancakes? YES, you can! And these pumpkin pancakes are delicious. You can make good-for-you pancakes without flour, and you're going to love them. They're a bit more delicate than the pancakes you're accustomed to so be sure the first side is fully cooked before you flip them.

Prep time: 5 min. • Cook time: 15 min. • Yield: Six 4-inch pancakes; 2 servings

2 large eggs

1/3 cup canned or cooked pumpkin purée (not pie filling)

2 tablespoons sunflower seed butter, almond butter, or other nut butter, unsweetened

Stevia or monk fruit sweetener, to equal 1/2 to 1 tablespoon sugar

3/4 teaspoon pumpkin pie spice

1/4 teaspoon baking powder

2 to 3 tablespoons pecans, chopped

Coconut oil cooking spray or coconut oil, for the pan

Put all of the ingredients in a medium bowl and whisk together until fully blended.

Heat a nonstick skillet over medium heat. Spray the pan with the coconut oil spray or lightly brush with coconut oil. Pour about 3 tablespoons of the batter into the preheated skillet to make a 4-inch pancake. Cook until the edges begin to brown and bubbles on the top begin to burst. Flip and cook until done. Repeat with the remaining batter.

Notes

Use care when flipping the pancakes. If the spatula doesn't slide under the edge of the pancake, it is probably not ready to flip. You can use two spatulas to make it easier to flip. Don't overcrowd the pan; it makes flipping tricky. Using a nonstick pan makes cooking easier.

(recipe continues)

If you don't have pumpkin pie spice, combine ½ teaspoon ground cinnamon, ⅛ teaspoon ground nutmeg, ⅛ teaspoon ground allspice, and a hefty pinch of ground ginger.

Chicken Piccata

This favorite Italian meal is easy to prepare. The word "piccata" refers to a cooking method for meat or fish in which the food is thinly sliced, sautéed, and served in a sauce containing lemon juice, butter, and capers. Serve on top of zoodles or cauliflower rice for a complete meal.

Prep time: 20 min. • Cook time: 15 min. • Yield: 4 servings

4 chicken breasts, boneless and skinless

1 teaspoon Celtic or pink Himalayan salt

½ teaspoon freshly ground black pepper

4 tablespoons almond flour

1 tablespoon olive oil

1 tablespoon ghee (see page 57) or pasture-raised butter

½ cup Chicken Bone Broth (page 179)

¼ cup fresh lemon juice

1 tablespoon lemon zest

¼ cup capers, drained and rinsed

¼ cup parsley, coarsely chopped

Place the chicken breasts between two sheets of plastic wrap. Using a meat mallet or the bottom of a skillet, pound the chicken to ¼-inch thickness. Sprinkle each breast with the salt and pepper and roll in the almond flour. Don't worry about any bare spots.

Heat a large skillet over medium-high heat and add the oil and ghee. Brown the chicken on both sides, about 3 to 4 minutes per side. Transfer the chicken to a plate and set aside. Add the bone broth, lemon juice, lemon zest, capers, and parsley to the pan. Stir, scraping up brown bits and incorporating into the sauce.

Place the chicken breasts back into the skillet and bring to a boil.

Immediately reduce the heat to low, cover, and simmer 8 to 10 minutes, or until the chicken is cooked through. Plate the chicken and spoon the sauce on top. Serve with cauliflower rice or steamed spinach.

Chicken Saltimbocca

Saltimbocca is an Italian dish also popular in southern Switzerland, Spain, and Greece. It is traditionally made with veal that is wrapped with prosciutto and sage. This recipe is also delicious made with turkey cutlets. You can slice a boneless turkey breast into cutlets or buy turkey cutlets ready to cook.

Prep time: 15 min. • Cook time: 25 min. • Yield: 4 servings

4 chicken breasts, boneless and skinless

½ teaspoon freshly ground black pepper

½ to 1 teaspoon garlic powder or granules

8 fresh sage leaves

3 ounces nitrate- and nitrite-free prosciutto (about 8 thin slices)

1 tablespoon olive oil

1 cup Chicken Bone Broth (page 179)

2 tablespoons ghee (see page 57) or pasture-raised butter

Place the chicken breasts between two sheets of plastic wrap. Using a meat mallet or the bottom of a skillet, pound the chicken to ¼-inch thickness. Sprinkle each breast with the pepper and garlic powder. Put 3 or 4 sage leaves on top of each breast and then wrap 2 slices of prosciutto crosswise over each piece to hold the sage in place.

Heat the oil in a large skillet over medium heat and brown the chicken on both sides, about 3 to 4 minutes per side. Transfer the chicken to a platter and tent with foil to keep warm.

Add the broth to the skillet and simmer for 4 to 5 minutes, or until reduced by about half, scraping up any brown bits to deglaze the pan.

(recipe continues)

Add the ghee and stir until melted and the sauce is creamy. Return the chicken to the skillet to heat through and serve, spooning the sauce over the chicken. Serve with cauliflower rice or steamed spinach.

Note
Prosciutto is naturally salty, so you won't need additional salt in this recipe.

Chicken Wraps with Tahini Lime Dressing

Tahini is roasted sesame seed butter often used in Middle Eastern cooking. If you like sesame seeds, you'll love tahini. It does tend to separate, so be sure to mix it well before using. If you store it in the pantry upside down, it'll be easier to blend. This dressing is also great on salads.

Prep time: 10 min. • Yield: 4 servings

For the Tahini Lime Dressing (serves 6; makes ¾ cup)

⅓ cup tahini, blended until smooth

1 garlic clove, very finely minced

2 tablespoons fresh lime juice (about ½ lime)

1 tablespoon olive oil

¼ teaspoon Celtic or pink Himalayan salt, plus more as needed

4 to 5 tablespoons lukewarm water

For the Lettuce Wraps

4 to 5 ounces rotisserie chicken, shredded

1 small carrot, shredded

4 cherry tomatoes cut in quarters, or about ½ cup plum tomatoes, diced

1 Persian cucumber or 3- to 4-inch piece English cucumber, thinly sliced or diced (about ½ cup)

2 tablespoons cilantro, coarsely chopped (optional)

4 large green leaf, butter lettuce, Bibb lettuce, romaine, or other lettuce leaves

Celtic or pink Himalayan salt and freshly ground black pepper to taste

Make the dressing: In a blender or food processor, add the tahini, garlic, lime juice, oil, and salt. Add the water a tablespoon at a time until the desired consistency is reached.

Make the wraps: In a small bowl, mix the chicken, carrot, tomatoes, cucumber, and cilantro (if using). Add 2 tablespoons of the tahini lime dressing and toss together. Scoop the chicken salad onto the lettuce leaves and top with the salt and pepper, if desired. Roll up like a burrito.

Note

You can also enjoy these as lettuce cups if you prefer to eat them with a fork.

Dijon Chicken Breasts with Artichoke Hearts and Sundried Tomatoes

Prep time: 15 min. • Cook time: 25 min. • Yield: 4 servings

4 chicken breasts or thighs, boneless and skinless

1 teaspoon Celtic or pink Himalayan salt

1/2 teaspoon freshly ground black pepper

1 tablespoon avocado oil

2 tablespoons ghee (see page 57) or pasture-raised butter

1 cup Chicken Bone Broth (page 179)

3 garlic cloves, minced

1 tablespoon Dijon mustard

1 (14-ounce) can artichoke hearts in water, drained and halved

1/2 cup sundried tomatoes, sliced (dry sundried tomatoes, not packed in oil)

Season the chicken breasts with salt and pepper. Heat the oil and ghee in a large skillet over medium-high heat and brown the chicken, about 3 to 4 minutes per side. Remove the chicken from the skillet and set on a plate.

In the same skillet, whisk together the bone broth, garlic, and mustard, scraping up any brown bits to deglaze the pan. Add the artichoke

(recipe continues)

hearts and sundried tomatoes, stir, and return the chicken breasts to the skillet, spooning the sauce over them. Cover, reduce the heat to low, and simmer 15 to 20 minutes, or until the chicken is cooked through.

To serve, spoon the sauce over the chicken. Serve with cauliflower rice or steamed spinach.

Popeye Spinach Power Bowl

This yummy spinach salad bowl is simple and satisfying. It's easy to put together with prepared foods already in the fridge: rotisserie chicken or deli turkey, precooked bacon, and a hard-boiled egg. And by all means use the extra dressing for salads, a sauce, or a marinade.

Prep time: 15 min. • Yield: 8 servings

For the Bowl

1 cup or more cauliflower rice

1 cup or more baby spinach

3 to 4 ounces rotisserie chicken, shredded, or 3 to 4 ounces nitrate-, nitrite-, and sugar-free deli turkey, sliced

1 hard-boiled egg, diced

1 slice nitrate-, nitrite-, and sugar-free turkey or pork bacon, cooked and diced

4 or 5 white or cremini mushrooms, sliced

A few slices of red onion

3 or 4 cherry tomatoes, cut in half

For the Sweet Onion Dressing
(serves 8 servings; makes a little more than 1 cup)

1/2 medium Vidalia, Maui, or other sweet onion

1/2 cup olive oil

2 tablespoons red wine vinegar

Stevia or monk fruit sweetener, to equal 3 to 4 tablespoons sugar

1/2 teaspoons dry mustard

1/2 teaspoon garlic powder

1/2 teaspoon Celtic or pink Himalayan salt

1/4 teaspoon freshly ground black pepper

2 to 3 teaspoons poppy seeds (optional)

Assemble the bowl: Place the cauliflower rice in a bowl and top with the spinach, chicken, egg, bacon, mushrooms, onion, and tomatoes.

Make the dressing: Cut off the top and bottom of the onion. Place the onion in a microwave-safe dish and make several slits in the onion's sides with a knife. Add a ½-inch of water to the dish, cover, and microwave for 4 minutes to soften the onion. Pour off the water, uncover, and set aside to cool completely.

When cool, cut the onion into several pieces and place in a blender or food processor. Add the oil, vinegar, stevia, mustard, garlic powder, salt, pepper, and poppy seeds (if using) and blend until smooth and creamy. Taste and adjust sweetness and salt to taste.

Toss the salad bowl with 1 tablespoon of the dressing and serve.

Notes

Store unused dressing in a closed container in the refrigerator for up to 2 weeks. Use as a salad dressing or a sauce or marinade for chicken.

Start with less sweetener than you think you'll need. A little goes a long way. When you taste the dressing you can determine if it needs more sweetness.

Pumpkin Chili

Pumpkin in chili? Yes! It adds an earthy richness to the chili along with fiber, vitamins, and minerals. So often when we think pumpkin, we think of desserts, but pumpkin adds a lot to savory recipes, too.

Prep time: 20 min. • Cook time: 35 min. • Yield: 4 to 6 servings

2 tablespoons olive oil

1 green bell pepper, diced

1 onion, diced

2 garlic cloves, minced

1/2 cup Italian parsley, coarsely chopped

1 pound ground turkey

1 to 2 tablespoons chili powder

1 teaspoon cumin

1 teaspoon Celtic or pink Himalayan salt

1/2 teaspoon freshly ground black pepper

1 (15-ounce) can diced tomatoes, drained

1 (15-ounce) can pumpkin (not pie filling)

2 cups Chicken Bone Broth (page 179)

1/4 cup fresh cilantro, chopped (optional)

1/4 cup red onion, chopped (optional)

Heat the oil in a deep skillet or Dutch oven over medium heat and sauté the bell pepper and onion for 5 minutes. Stir in the garlic, parsley, and ground turkey and sauté over medium-high heat until the turkey is browned. When the meat is fully cooked stir in the chili powder, cumin, salt, and pepper.

Add the diced tomatoes, pumpkin, and bone broth. Bring the mixture to a boil, reduce the heat to low, and simmer, covered, for 15 minutes. Uncover and cook 15 minutes more, or to desired consistency. Serve with the cilantro and onion, if desired.

Note

I love to spoon a serving of this chili into half of a roasted spaghetti squash. You can also add a scoop of cauliflower rice to a bowl of chili.

Shrimp with Rosemary and Pancetta

This is a classic shrimp dish from southern Italy, enhanced with pancetta and rosemary. It's aromatic and quick and easy to make. Reducing the bone broth and tomatoes makes an amazing pan sauce!

Prep time: 10 min. • Cook time: 20 min. • Yield: 4 servings

1 ounce pancetta (about 1 slice) or 2 slices of bacon, diced

1 tablespoon olive oil

2 garlic cloves, very thinly sliced

2 plum tomatoes, seeded and diced

1½ teaspoons fresh rosemary, finely chopped

1 cup Chicken Bone Broth (page 179)

¼ teaspoon freshly ground black pepper

1½ pounds large shrimp, peeled and deveined

2 tablespoons ghee (see page 57) or pasture-raised butter

Celtic or pink Himalayan salt to taste (optional)

In a large skillet over medium-high heat, sauté the pancetta until browned and crispy. Remove from the pan and set aside on a plate lined with a paper towel. In the same pan add the olive oil, garlic, tomatoes, and rosemary and sauté for 3 minutes. Add the bone broth and pepper and simmer, stirring occasionally until the broth is reduced by half. Add the shrimp and cook on medium heat for 8 to 10 minutes to cook through. Add the ghee and pancetta and mix all the ingredients together until the ghee is fully melted into the sauce. Taste and salt if needed.

Serve over cauliflower rice with the pan sauce.

Note

Both pancetta and bacon are salty, so you probably don't need any additional salt in this recipe.

It's true that making fresh meals with clean, natural foods isn't as easy as zapping a container of frozen lasagna from the grocery store. However, there are plenty of meals you can toss together fast when life is hectic. Here are some of my favorites:

- A large garden salad dressed with olive oil and vinegar or lemon plus sautéed veggies and a protein of your choice.
- Any of my broth loading soups with added protein.
- Rotisserie chicken and a garden salad dressed with olive oil and vinegar or lemon.
- Smoked salmon with onions, capers, and lemon and one or two vegetables on the side.
- Egg salad or tuna salad dressed with 1 tablespoon avocado mayo and ¼ avocado, served on a bed of lettuce with sliced tomatoes and cucumbers.
- Spiralized zucchini with a simple Bolognese sauce.
- Cauliflower "fried rice" topped with a protein of your choice.
- A turkey, beef, or bison burger in a lettuce wrap with avocado mayo as a condiment.
- Deli turkey in a lettuce wrap with ½ avocado or avocado mayo.
- A bowl of homemade chili (see page 228) served over cauliflower rice.
- A chef salad with deli turkey, rotisserie chicken, hard-boiled eggs, or a combination of proteins, served with ½ avocado or dressed with olive oil and vinegar or lemon.
- A large bowl of sautéed veggies with a protein of your choice.

Shrimp with cocktail sauce (use sugar-free ketchup and
add fresh horseradish), served with a salad or veggies.

It's very easy to come up with many other post-cleanse meals.
Simply stick to the template on pages 87–91, and you're good to
go. And here's another tip: don't forget leftovers because they're
the easiest grab-and-go meal of all!

P.S.—Tell Me About Your Cleanse!

I know how this cleanse changed my life for the better, and now I'd
love to hear what it does for you. So take a minute and share your
cleanse story with me and my community!

The official hashtag is #drkellyanncleanse. If you add this hashtag
to your social media posts, my team and others looking for inspiration will be able to view your post and connect with you. You can
search this hashtag on Instagram, Facebook, and Twitter and see what
is being shared about the diet, including fun recipe ideas.

In addition, check out my Facebook page at facebook.com/groups
/DrKellyannsCleanse. I have a huge and wonderful community of
people who love to share recipes, tips, and inspiration, and they'd love
to meet you.

Follow me on Twitter @DrKellyann and on Instagram
@DrKellyannPetrucci.

Carb Counter: Whether you want to stay moderately low-carb or go
full-out keto, it's important to know the carb counts of the foods you
choose. Here's a handy chart (see pages 232 through 236) that tells you
how many carbs—and, more important, how many *net* carbs—there
are in different fruits, veggies, nuts, and seeds.

NUTS AND SEEDS	SERVING SIZE	TOTAL CARBS (G)	FIBER (G)	NET CARBS (G)
Almonds	¼ cup	11	6.5	4.5
Brazil Nuts	¼ cup	6	3.75	2.25
Cashews	¼ cup	15	1.65	13.35
Chestnuts	¼ cup	17.5	0	17.5
Chia Seeds	2 Tbsps	10.5	8.5	2
Flaxseeds	2 Tbsps	7.25	6.75	2.5
Hazelnuts	¼ cup	8.5	4.85	3.65
Hemp Seeds	¼ cup	4.35	4	0.35
Macadamia Nuts	¼ cup	7	4.3	2.7
Peanuts	¼ cup	8	4.75	3.25
Pecans	¼ cup	7	4.8	2.2
Pine Nuts	¼ cup	6.5	1.85	4.65
Pistachios	¼ cup	13.5	5.5	8
Poppy Seeds	2 Tbsps	7	5	2
Pumpkin Seeds	¼ cup	5.5	3	2.5
Sesame Seeds	2 Tbsps	5.75	3	2.75
Sunflower Seeds	¼ cup	10	4.3	5.7
Walnuts	¼ cup	7	3.35	3.65

FRUITS	SERVING SIZE	TOTAL CARBS (G)	FIBER (G)	NET CARBS (G)
Apricots	½ cup	11	2	9
Bananas	½ cup	23	2.6	20.4
Blackberries	½ cup	9.6	5.3	4.3
Blueberries	½ cup	14	2.4	11.6
Boysenberries	½ cup	12	5.3	6.7
Cantaloupes	½ cup	8.2	0.9	7.3
Cherimoyas	½ cup	18	3	15
Cherries (sour)	½ cup	12	1.6	10.4
Cherries (sweet)	½ cup	16	2.1	13.9
Clementines	½ cup	12	1.7	9.3
Coconut	½ cup	15	9	6

FRUITS	SERVING SIZE	TOTAL CARBS (G)	FIBER (G)	NET CARBS (G)
Cranberries	½ cup	12	3.6	8.4
Currants	½ cup	14	4.3	97
Elderberries	½ cup	18	7	11
Figs	½ cup	19	2.9	16.1
Gooseberries	½ cup	10	4.3	5.7
Granny Smith Apple	½ cup	14	2.4	11.6
Grapes	½ cup	18	0.9	17.
Grapefruit	½ cup	8.2	0	8.2
Guava	½ cup	14	5.4	8.6
Honeydew	½ cup	9.1	0.8	8.3
Huckleberries	½ cup	8.7	0	8.7
Jackfruits	½ cup	23	1.5	21.5
Jujubes	½ cup	20	0	20
Kiwis	½ cup	15	3	12
Kumquats	½ cup	16	6.5	9.5
Lemons	½ cup	9.3	2.8	6.5
Limes	½ cup	11	2.8	8.2
Longans	½ cup	15	1.1	13.9
Loquats	½ cup	12	1.7	10.3
Mangoes	½ cup	15	1.6	13.4
Mulberries	½ cup	9.8	1.7	8.1
Nectarines	½ cup	11	1.7	9.3
Papayas	½ cup	11	1.7	9.3
Passionfruit	½ cup	23	10	13
Peaches	½ cup	14	0.6	13.4
Pears	½ cup	15	3.1	11.9
Pineapple	½ cup	13	1.4	11.6
Plantains	½ cup	32	2.3	29.7
Plums	½ cup	11	1.4	9.6
Pomegranate	½ cup	19	4	15
Pummelos	½ cup	9.6	1	8.6
Quinces	½ cup	15	1.9	13.1

FRUITS	SERVING SIZE	TOTAL CARBS (G)	FIBER (G)	NET CARBS (G)
Raspberries	½ cup	12	6.5	5.5
Rhubarb	½ cup	4.5	1.8	2.7
Star Fruit	½ cup	6.7	2.8	3.9
Strawberries	½ cup	7.7	2	5.7
Tangerines	½ cup	13	1.8	11.2
Watermelon	½ cup	7.6	0.4	7.2

VEGETABLES	SERVING SIZE	TOTAL CARBS (G)	FIBER (G)	NET CARBS (G)
Acorn Squash (raw)	1 cup	15	2.1	12.9
Arrowroot (raw)	1 cup	16	1.6	14.4
Artichoke Hearts (canned)	½ cup	11	5.4	5.6
Arugula (raw)	1 cup	0.8	0.4	0.4
Asparagus (raw)	1 cup	5.2	2.8	2.4
Avocados (raw)	1 cup	13	10	3
Beet Greens (raw)	1 cup	1.7	1.4	0.3
Beets (raw)	1 cup	13	3.8	9.2
Bell Peppers, Green (raw)	1 cup	4.3	1.6	2.7
Bell Peppers, Red (raw)	1 cup	5.6	1.9	3.7
Bell Peppers, Yellow (raw)	1 cup	6.3	0.9	5.4
Broccoli (raw)	1 cup	6	2.4	3.6
Broccoli Rabe (raw)	1 cup	1.1	1.1	0
Brussels Sprouts (raw)	1 cup	7.9	3.3	4.6
Butternut Squash (raw)	1 cup	16	2.8	13.2
Cabbage, Green (raw)	1 cup	4.1	1.8	2.3
Cabbage, Red (raw)	1 cup	5.2	1.5	3.7
Carrots (raw)	½ cup	9.6	2.8	6.8

VEGETABLES	SERVING SIZE	TOTAL CARBS (G)	FIBER (G)	NET CARBS (G)
Cassava (raw)	¼ cup	19.5	0.9	18.6
Cauliflower (raw)	1 cup	5.3	2.1	3.2
Celery (raw)	1 cup	3	1.6	1.4
Celery Root (raw)	1 cup	14	2.8	11.2
Chile Peppers (raw)	½ cup	8.8	1.5	7.3
Chinese Cabbage (raw)	1 cup	1.5	0.7	0.8
Chives (raw)	2 tbs	0.2	0.2	0
Collard Greens (raw)	1 cup	2	1.4	0.6
Cucumbers (raw) with peel	1 cup	3.8	0.6	3.2
Daikon Radish (raw)	1 cup	4.8	1.9	2.9
Eggplant (raw)	1 cup	4.8	2.5	2.3
Endive (raw)	1 cup	1.6	1.6	0
Fennel (raw bulb)	1 cup	6.4	2.7	3.7
Ginger Root (raw)	2 Tbsp	2.15	0.25	1.9
Green Beans (raw)	1 cup	7	2.7	4.3
Green Onions (raw)	1 cup	7	2.6	4.4
Jalapeño Peppers (raw)	1 cup	5.9	2.5	3.4
Jicama (raw)	1 cup	11	6.4	4.6
Kale (raw)	1 cup	1.4	0.6	0.8
Kohlrabies (raw)	1 cup	8.4	4.9	3.5
Leeks (raw)	1 cup	13	1.6	11.4
Lettuce, Green Leaf (raw)	1 cup	1	0.5	0.5
Lettuce, Romaine (raw)	1 cup	1.6	1	0.6
Mushrooms, Portobello (raw)	1 cup	3.3	1.1	2.2
Mushrooms, White (raw)	1 cup	2.3	0.7	1.6
Mustard Greens (raw)	1 cup	2.6	1.8	0.8

VEGETABLES	SERVING SIZE	TOTAL CARBS (G)	FIBER (G)	NET CARBS (G)
Napa Cabbage (raw)	1 cup	1.5	0.7	0.8
Okra (raw)	1 cup	7.5	3.2	4.3
Olives (canned)	10 olives	3	1	2
Onions, White (raw)	1 cup	15	2.7	12.3
Parsnips (raw)	½ cup	12	6.5	5.5
Peas, green (raw)	1 cup	21	8.3	12.7
Potatoes, Red (raw)	½ cup	12	1.3	10.7
Potatoes, White (raw)	½ cup	12	1.8	10.2
Potatoes, Yellow (raw)	½ cup	12	2	10
Pumpkin (raw)	1 cup	7.5	0.6	6.9
Radicchio (raw)	1 cup	1.8	0.4	1.4
Radishes (raw)	1 cup	3.9	1.9	2
Onions, red (raw)	1 cup	16	2	14
Rutabaga (raw)	1 cup	12	3.2	8.8
Shallots (raw)	.25 cup	6.8	1.2	5.6
Spaghetti Squash (raw)	1 cup	7	1.5	5.5
Spinach (raw)	1 cup	1.1	0.7	0.4
Summer Squash (raw)	½ cup	3.4	1.1	2.3
Sweet Potatoes (raw)	½ cup	13.5	2	11.5
Swiss Chard (raw)	1 cup	1.4	0.6	0.8
Tomatoes (raw)	1 cup	7	2.2	4.8
Turnip Greens (raw)	1 cup	3.9	1.8	2.1
Turnips (raw)	1 cup	8.4	2.3	6.1
Watercress (raw)	1 cup	0.4	0.2	0.2
Yams (raw)	½ cup	21	3.1	17.9
Zucchini (raw)	1 cup	3.5	1.1	2.4

Notes

Chapter 2

1. John Berardi, "Chances Are, You've Got a Deficiency," *Precision Nutrition*, precisionnutrition.com/balanced-diet-isnt-enough.

2. B. Misner, "Food Alone May Not Provide Sufficient Micronutrients for Preventing Deficiency," *Journal of the International Society of Sports Nutrition*, June 5, 2006, 3(1): 51–55: ncbi.nlm.nih.gov/pmc/articles/PMC2129155/.

3. J. Bae et al., "Bog Blueberry Anthocyanins Alleviate Photoaging in Ultraviolet-B Irradiation-Induced Human Dermal Fibroblasts," *Molecular Nutrition & Food Research*, June 9, 2009, 53(6): 726–38; onlinelibrary.wiley.com/doi /abs/10.1002/mnfr.200800245.

4. L.Wang and G. D. Stoner, "Anthocyanins and Their Role in Cancer Prevention," *Cancer Letters*, October 8, 2008, 269(2): 281–90; ncbi.nlm.nih.gov/pmc /articles/PMC2582525/.

5. M. Riaz et al., "The Role of Anthocyanins in Obesity and Diabetes," *Anthocyanins and Human Health: Biomolecular and Therapeutic Aspects*, April 12, 2016, 109–23; link.springer.com/chapter/10.1007/978-3-319-26456-1_8.

6. M. El-Sayed et al., "Dietary Sources of Lutein and Zeaxanthin Carotenoids and Their Role in Eye Health," *Nutrients*, April 2013, 5(4): 1169–85; ncbi.nlm .nih.gov/pmc/articles/PMC3705341/.

7. P. Chaudhary et al., "Bioactivities of Phytochemicals Present in Tomato," *Journal of Food Science and Technology*, August 2018, 55(8): 2833–49; ncbi.nlm .nih.gov/pubmed/30065393.

8. X. Li and J. Xu, "Lycopene Supplement and Blood Pressure: an Updated Meta-Analysis of Intervention Trials," *Nutrients*, September 2013, 5(9): 3696–3712; ncbi.nlm.nih.gov/pmc/articles/PMC3798929/.

9. K. Jade, "Impressive Lycopene Benefits: Reduces Stroke Risk by 59%," *University Health News Daily*, March 7, 2018; universityhealthnews.com/daily /heart-health/the-brainiest-reason-to-eat-more-tomatoes-lycopene-benefits -brain-health-in-more-ways-than-one/.

10. Z. Ungvari et al., "Mitochondrial Protection by Resveratrol," *Exercise and Sport Sciences Reviews*, July 1, 2012, 39(3): 128–32; ncbi.nlm.nih.gov/pmc /articles/PMC3123408/.

11. T. Suzuki and H. Hara, "Role of Flavonoids in Intestinal Tight Junction

Regulation," *Journal of Nutritional Biochemistry*, May 2011, 22(5): 401–08; sciencedirect.com/science/article/pii/S0955286310001877.

12. S. Agarwal, "Comparison of Prevalence of Inadequate Nutrient Intake Based on Body Weight Status of Adults in the United States: an Analysis of NHANES 2001–2008," *Journal of the American College of Nutrition*, 2015, 34(2): 126–34; ncbi.nlm.nih.gov/pubmed/?term=Comparison+of+Prevalence +of+Inadequate+Nutrient+Intake+Based+on+Body+Weight+Status+of+Adults +in+the+United+States%3A+An+Analysis+of+NHANES+2001-2008.

13. M. Via, "The Malnutrition of Obesity: Micronutrient Deficiencies That Promote Diabetes," *ISRN Endocrinology*, March 15, 2012 (online); ncbi.nlm.nih .gov/pmc/articles/PMC3313629/.

14. Yan Jiang et al., "A Sucrose-Enriched Diet Promotes Tumorigenesis in Mammary Gland in Part Through the 12-Lipoxygenase Pathway," *Cancer Research*, January 2016 (online), cancerres.aacrjournals.org/content/76/1/24.

15. J. M. Wojcicki et al., "Increased Cellular Aging by 3 Years of Age in Latino, Preschool Children Who Consume More Sugar-Sweetened Beverages: a Pilot Study," *Childhood Obesity*, April 2018, 14(3): 149–57; ncbi.nlm.nih.gov /pubmed/29148828.

16. J. Norris, "Sugared Soda Consumption, Cell Aging Associated in New Study," UCSF News Center, October 16, 2014; ucsf.edu/news/2014/10/119431 /sugared-soda-consumption-cell-aging-associated-new-study.

17. M. K. Caldow et al., "Glycine Supplementation During Calorie Restriction Accelerates Fat Loss and Protects Against Further Muscle Loss in Obese Mice," *Clinical Nutrition*, October 2016, 35(5): 1118–26; ncbi.nlm.nih.gov /pubmed/26431812.

18. M. El-Hafidi et al., "Glycine Increases Insulin Sensitivity and Glutathione Biosynthesis and Protects Against Oxidative Stress in a Model of Sucrose-Induced Insulin Resistance," *Oxidative Medicine and Cellular Longevity*, February 21, 2018 (online); ncbi.nlm.nih.gov/pmc/articles/PMC5841105/.

19. M. C. Gannon et al., "The Metabolic Response to Ingested Glycine," *American Journal of Clinical Nutrition*, December 2002, 76(6): 1302–07; ncbi.nlm.nih .gov/pubmed/12450897; see also Pamela Schoenfeld, *The Collagen Diet* (Berkeley, CA: Ulysses Press, 2018).

20. E. Meléndez-Hevia et al, "A Weak Link in Metabolism: The Metabolic Capacity for Glycine Biosynthesis Does Not Satisfy the Need for Collagen Synthesis," *Journal of Biosciences*, December 2009, 34(6): 853–72; ias.ac.in/article /fulltext/jbsc/034/06/0853-0872.

21. A. Howard et al, "Glycine Transporter GLYT1 Is Essential for Glycine-Mediated Protection of Human Intestinal Epithelial Cells Against Oxida-

tive Damage," *Journal of Physiology*, 2010, 588(6): 995–1009; ncbi.nlm.nih.gov /pmc/articles/PMC2849964/pdf/tjp0588-0995.pdf.

22. E. Proksch et al., "Oral Intake of Specific Bioactive Collagen Peptides Reduces Skin Wrinkles and Increases Dermal Matrix Synthesis," *Skin Pharmacology and Physiology*, 2014, 27(3): 113–19; ncbi.nlm.nih.gov/pubmed/24401291.

23. L. Genser et al., "Increased Jejunal Permeability in Human Obesity Is Revealed by a Lipid Challenge and Is Linked to Inflammation and Type 2 Diabetes," *Journal of Pathology*, October 2018, 246(2): 217–30; ncbi.nlm.nih.gov /pubmed/29984492.

24. M. C. Hochberg et al., "Combined Chondroitin Sulfate and Glucosamine for Painful Knee Osteoarthritis: a Multicentre, Randomised, Double-Blind, Non-Inferiority Trial Versus Celecoxib," *Annals of the Rheumatic Diseases*, 2016, 75(1): 37–44; ard.bmj.com/content/75/1/37.

25. J. Scala et al., "Effect of Daily Gelatin Ingestion on Human Scalp Hair," *Nutrition Reports International*, January 1976, 13(6): 579–92; researchgate .net/publication/279548216_Effect_of_daily_gelatin_ingestion_on_human _scalp_hair.

26. T. L. Tyson, "The Effect of Gelatin on Fragile Finger Nails," *Journal of Investigative Dermatology*, May 1950, 14(5): 323–25; jidonline.org/article/S0022 -202X(15)50492-2/abstract.

27. Alanna Collen, *10% Human* (New York: HarperCollins, 2015).

28. P. Gonçalves and F. Martel, "Butyrate and Colorectal Cancer: The Role of Butyrate Transport," *Current Drug Metabolism*, November 2013, 14(9): 994– 1008; ncbi.nlm.nih.gov/pubmed/24160296.

29. Z. Gao et al., "Butyrate Improves Insulin Sensitivity and Increases Energy Expenditure in Mice," *Diabetes*, July 2009, 58(7): 1509–17; diabetes.diabetes journals.org/content/58/7/1509.long.

30. Q. Zhang et al., "Beetroot Red (Betanin) Inhibits Vinyl Carbamate- and Benzo(a)pyrene-Induced Lung Tumorigenesis Through Apoptosis," *Molecular Carcinogenesis*, March 27, 2012 (online); onlinelibrary.wiley.com/doi /full/10.1002/mc.21907.

31. G. J. Kapadia et al., "Chemoprevention of DMBA-Induced UV-B Promoted, NOR-1-Induced TPA Promoted Skin Carcinogenesis, and DEN-Induced Phenobarbital Promoted Liver Tumors in Mice by Extract of Beetroot," *Pharmacological Research*, February 2003, 47(2): 141–48; ncbi.nlm.nih.gov /pubmed/12543062.

32. M. J. Turokey, "Molecular Targets of Luteolin in Cancer," *European Journal of Cancer Prevention*, December 2, 2015 (online); ncbi.nlm.nih.gov/pmc/articles /PMC4885545/.

33. B. Sung et al., "Role of Apigenin in Cancer Prevention via the Induction of Apoptosis and Sutophagy," *Journal of Cancer Prevention*, December 2016, 21(4): 216–26; ncbi.nlm.nih.gov/pubmed/28053955.

34. "Cruciferous Vegetables and Cancer Prevention," National Cancer Institute; cancer.gov/about-cancer/causes-prevention/risk/diet/cruciferous-vegetables -fact-sheet.

35. A. J. Cooper, "A Prospective Study of the Association Between Quantity and Variety of Fruit and Vegetable Intake and Incident Type 2 Diabetes," *Diabetes Care*, June 2012, 35(6): 1293–1300; care.diabetesjournals.org /content/35/6/1293.

36. F. L. Büchner et al., "Variety in Fruit and Vegetable Consumption and the Risk of Lung Cancer in the European Prospective Investigation into Cancer and Nutrition," *Cancer Epidemiology, Biomarkers & Prevention*, September 2010, 19(9): 2278–86; ncbi.nlm.nih.gov/pubmed/20807832.

37. C. D. Gardner et al., "Comparison of the Atkins, Zone, Ornish, and LEARN Diets for Change in Weight and Related Risk Factors Among Overweight Premenopausal Women: The A to Z Weight Loss Study: A Randomized Trial," *Journal of the American Medical Association*, March 2007, 297(9): 969–77; jamanetwork.com/journals/jama/fullarticle/205916.

38. T. Jönsson et al., "Beneficial Effects of a Paleolithic Diet on Cardiovascular Risk Factors in Type 2 Diabetes: A Randomized Cross-Over Pilot Study," *Cardiovascular Diabetology*, 2009; ncbi.nlm.nih.gov/pubmed/?term=Beneficial +effects+of+a+Paleolithic+diet+on+cardiovascular+risk+factors+in+type+2 + diabetes%3A+a+randomized+cross-over+pilot+study.

39. "Low Glycaemic Index or Low Glycaemic Load Diets for Overweight and Obesity," Cochrane Collaboration, 2007; cochrane.org/CD005105/ENDOC _low-glycaemic-index-or-low-glycaemic-load-diets-for-overweight-and -obesity.

Chapter 3

1. K. Nikos-Rose, "Sugar-Sweetened Beverages Are Harmful to Health and May Be Addictive, Researchers Suggest," medicalxpress, November 20, 2018; medicalxpress.com/news/2018-11-sugar-sweetened-beverages-health -addictive.html.

2. A. G. Walton, "Why Oreos Are as Addictive as Cocaine to Your Brain," *Forbes*, October 16, 2013; forbes.com/sites/alicegwalton/2013/10/16/why-your-brain -treats-oreos-like-a-drug/#52b22b35ab00.

3. Q. Xiang-Yang et al., "Mogrosides Extract from *Siraitia Grosvenori* Scavenges Free Radicals in Vitro and Lowers Oxidative Stress, Serum Glucose, and Lipid

Levels in Alloxan-Induced Diabetic Mice," *Nutrition Research*, April 2008, 28(4): 278–84; sciencedirect.com/science/article/pii/S0271531708000365.

4. X. Zhang et al., "Effects of Mogrosides on High-Fat-Diet-Induced Obesity and Nonalcoholic Fatty Liver Disease in Mice," *Molecules*, 2018, 23(8); mdpi .com/1420-3049/23/8/1894.

5. B. Sun et al., "Anti-Obesity Effects of Mogrosides Extracted from the Fruits of *Siraitia Grosvenorii* (Cucurbitaceae)," *African Journal of Pharmacy and Pharmacology*, May 2012, 6(20): 1492–1501; academicjournals.org/journal/AJPP /article-abstract/088D6DA28337.

6. C. Zou et al., "Mogroside IIIE Attenuates Gestational Diabetes Mellitus Through Activating of AMPK Signaling Pathway in Mice," *Journal of Pharmacological Sciences*, November 2018, 138(3): 161–66; sciencedirect.com /science/article/pii/S1347861318301798?via%3Dihub.

7. C. Liu et al., "A Natural Food Sweetener with Anti-Pancreatic Cancer Properties," *Oncogenesis*, April 2016, 5(4): e217; ncbi.nlm.nih.gov/pmc/articles /PMC4848839/.

8. C. Liu et al., "Antiproliferative Activity of Triterpene Glycoside Nutrient from Monk Fruit in Colorectal Cancer and Throat Cancer," *Nutrients*, 2016, 8(6): 360; mdpi.com/2072-6643/8/6/360/htm.

9. A. Li-ping, "Acute Toxicity and Mutagenicity of *Siraitia Grosvenorii* Extract in Mice," *Journal of Anhui Agricultural Sciences*, 2014; en.cnki.com.cn/Article_en /CJFDTotal-AHNY201403050.htm.

Chapter 4

1. "Black Pepper Fights Formation of Fat Cells," UPI, May 7, 2012; upi.com /Health_News/2012/05/07/Black-pepper-fights-formation-of-fat-cells/UPI -20801336435628/#ixzz1uHsvZGNI

2. "Green Tea Boosts Production of Detox Enzymes, Rendering Cancerous Chemicals Harmless," *Science Daily*, August 12, 2007; sciencedaily.com /releases/2007/08/070810194923.htm.

3. J. L. Davis, "The Health Benefits of Tea," WebMD; webmd.com/food-recipes /features/health-benefits-tea.

4. K. Diepvens et al., "Obesity and Thermogenesis Related to the Consumption of Caffeine, Ephedrine, Capsaicin, and Green Tea," *American Journal of Physiology*, January 1, 2007; physiology.org/doi/full/10.1152/ajpregu.00832.2005.

5. S. K. Katiyar et al., "Silymarin, a Flavonoid from Milk Thistle (*Silybum marianum L.*), Inhibits UV-Induced Oxidative Stress Through Targeting Infiltrating CD11b+ Cells in Mouse Skin," *Photochemistry and Photobiology*, November 28, 2007; onlinelibrary.wiley.com/doi/abs/10.1111/j.1751-1097.2007.00241.x.

6. F. S. Predes et al., "Antioxidative and in *Vitro* Antiproliferative Activity of *Arctium Lappa* Root Extracts," *BMC Complementary & Alternative Medicine*, March 23, 2011 (online); ncbi.nlm.nih.gov/pmc/articles/PMC3073957/.

7. K. Gonsalves, "Best Coffee News You'll Hear All Day," *Prevention*, January 13, 2014; prevention.com/food-nutrition/healthy-eating/a20465840/coffee-hydrates-like-water-study/.

8. "Coffee Compounds That Could Help Prevent Type 2 Diabetes Identified," *Science Daily*, December 2, 2015; sciencedaily.com/releases/2015/12/151202124610.htm.

9. J. Collingwood, "Coffee May Prevent Dementia," PsychCentral, October 8, 2018; psychcentral.com/lib/coffee-may-prevent-dementia.

10. N. Davis, "Coffee Cuts Risk of Dying from Stroke and Heart Disease, Study Suggests," *The Guardian*, July 10, 2017; theguardian.com/science/2017/jul/10/coffee-cuts-risk-of-dying-from-stroke-and-heart-disease-study-suggests.

11. V. E. Fernández-Elías et al., "Ingestion of a Moderately High Caffeine Dose Before Exercise Increases Postexercise Energy Expenditure," *International Journal of Sport Nutrition and Exercise Metabolism*, February 2015, 25(1): 46–53; ncbi.nlm.nih.gov/pubmed/24901809.

12. M. M. Schubert et al., "Caffeine Consumption Around an Exercise Bout: Effects on Energy Expenditure, Energy Intake, and Exercise Enjoyment," *Journal of Applied Physiology*, August 14, 2014, 117(7): 745–54; ncbi.nlm.nih.gov/pubmed/25123196.

13. M. J. Duncan et al., "Acute Caffeine Ingestion Enhances Strength Performance and Reduces Perceived Exertion and Muscle Pain Perception During Resistance Exercise," *European Journal of Sport Science*, 2013, 13(4): 392–99; ncbi.nlm.nih.gov/pubmed/23834545.

14. D. Harpaz et al., "Measuring Artificial Sweeteners Toxicity Using a Bioluminescent Bacterial Panel," *Molecules*, September 25, 2018 (online); see also "Artificial Sweeteners Have Toxic Effects on Gut Microbes," *Science Daily*, October 1, 2018; sciencedaily.com/releases/2018/10/181001101932.htm.

15. M. P. St-Onge et al., "Weight-Loss Diet That Includes Consumption of Medium-Chain Triacylglycerol Oil Leads to a Greater Rate of Weight and Fat Mass Loss Than Does Olive Oil," *American Journal of Clinical Nutrition*, March 2008, 87(3): 621–26; ncbi.nlm.nih.gov/pubmed/18326600.

16. M. P. St-Onge et al., "Medium-Chain Triglycerides Increase Energy Expenditure and Decrease Adiposity in Overweight Men," *Obesity Research*, March 2003, 11(3): 395–402; ncbi.nlm.nih.gov/pubmed/12634436.

Chapter 5

1. For a sampling of studies pertaining to grains and inflammation, see K. de Punder and L. Pruimboom, "The Dietary Intake of Wheat and Other Cereal Grains and Their Role in Inflammation," *Nutrients*, March 2013, 5(3): 771–87; ncbi.nlm.nih.gov/pmc/articles/PMC3705319/.

2. S. N. Mahmood and W. P. Bowe, "Diet and Acne Update: Carbohydrates Emerge as the Main Culprit," *Journal of Drugs in Dermatology*, April 2014, 13(4): 428–35; jddonline.com/articles/dermatology/S1545961614P0428X.

3. C. B. Ebbeling et al., "Effects of a Low Carbohydrate Diet on Energy Expenditure During Weight Loss Maintenance: Randomized Trial," *British Medical Journal*, November 14, 2018 (online), bmj.com/content/363/bmj.k4583; see also A. Pawlowski, "For Weight-Loss Maintenance, a Low-Carb Diet May Be Best," *Today*, November 14, 2018, today.com/health/weight-loss-maintenance-low-carb-diet-may-be-best-t142060.

4. J. Polivy et al., "The Effect of Deprivation on Food Cravings and Eating Behavior in Restrained and Unrestrained Eaters," *International Journal of Eating Disorders*, December 2005, 38(4): 301–09; onlinelibrary.wiley.com/doi/pdf/10.1002/eat.20195.

5. L. Tran et al., "Soy Extracts Suppressed Iodine Uptake and Stimulated the Production of Autoimmunogen in Rat Thyrocytes," *Experimental Biology and Medicine*, June 2013, 238(6): 623–30; ncbi.nlm.nih.gov/pubmed/23918874.

6. L. B. Bindels et al., "Resistant Starch Can Improve Insulin Sensitivity Independently of the Gut Microbiota," *Microbiome*, February 2017, 5(1): 12; ncbi.nlm.nih.gov/pubmed/28166818.

7. D. Shen et al., "Positive Effects of Resistant Starch Supplementation on Bowel Function in Healthy Adults: a Systematic Review and Meta-Analysis of Randomized Controlled Trials," *International Journal of Food Sciences and Nutrition*, March 2017, 68(2): 149–57; ncbi.nlm.nih.gov/pubmed/27593182.

8. X. Yang et al., "Resistant Starch Regulates Gut Microbiota: Structure, Biochemistry and Cell Signaling," *Cell Physiology and Biochemistry*, 2017, 42(1): 306–18; ncbi.nlm.nih.gov/pubmed/28535508.

9. C. H. Emilien et al., "Effect of Resistant Wheat Starch on Subjective Appetite and Food Intake in Healthy Adults," *Nutrition*, November–December 2017: 69–74; ncbi.nlm.nih.gov/pubmed/28935147.

10. J. A. Higgins, "Resistant Starch: Metabolic Effects and Potential Health Benefits," *Journal of AOAC International*, May–June 2004, 87(3): 761–68; ncbi.nlm.nih.gov/pubmed/15287677.

11. L. Wang et al., "Alcohol Consumption, Weight Gain, and Risk of Becoming Overweight in Middle-Aged and Older Women," *Archives of Internal Medicine*, March 8, 2010, 170(5): 453–61; europepmc.org/articles/PMC2837522.

12. D. W. Droste et al., "A Daily Glass of Red Wine Associated with Lifestyle Changes Independently Improves Blood Lipids in Patients with Carotid Arteriosclerosis: Results from a Randomized Controlled Trial," *Nutrition Journal*, 2013 (online); ncbi.nlm.nih.gov/pmc/articles/PMC3833853/.

Chapter 6

1. Intermountain Medical Center, "Study Finds Routine Periodic Fasting Is Good for Your Health, and Your Heart," news release, April 3, 2011, eurekalert .org/pub_releases/2011-04/imc-sfr033111.php.

2. K. Lee et al., "Biomarkers Related to Oxidative Stress and Obesity Among Volunteers Participating in the Fasting Program," *Cancer Research*, April 2004, 64(7); cancerres.aacrjournals.org/content/64/7_Supplement/113.4; see also, J. B. Johnson et al., "Alternate Day Calorie Restriction Improves Clinical Findings and Reduces Markers of Oxidative Stress and Inflammation in Overweight Adults with Moderate Asthma," *Free Radical Biology & Medicine*, March 1, 2007, 42(5): 665–74; ncbi.nlm.nih.gov/pubmed/17291990/.

3. J. Zhang et al., "Intermittent Fasting Protects Against Alzheimer's Disease Possibly Through Restoring Aquaporin-4 Polarity," *Frontiers in Molecular Neuroscience*, November 29, 2017 (online); ncbi.nlm.nih.gov/pubmed/29238290.

4. M. P. Mattson, "Energy Intake, Meal Frequency, and Health: a Neurobiological Perspective," *Annual Review of Nutrition* 2005, 25(1): 237–60; ncbi.nlm.nih .gov/pubmed/16011467.

5. University of Alabama at Birmingham, "Time-Restricted Feeding Study Shows Promise in Helping People Shed Body Fat," *Science Daily*, January 6, 2017; sciencedaily.com/releases/2017/01/170106113820.htm.

6. E. Betuel, "When You Eat Breakfast and Dinner Could Affect Your Levels of Body Fat," Yahoo News, August 31, 2018; news.yahoo.com/eat-breakfast -dinner-could-affect-164200986.html.

7. C. L. Goodrick et al., "Effects of Intermittent Feeding upon Growth and Life Span in Rats," *Gerontology*, 1982, no. 28: 233–41; karger.com/Article /Abstract/212538.

8. "Study: Daily Fasting Improves Health and Longevity in Male Mice," *Sci News*, September 12, 2018; sci-news.com/medicine/daily-fasting-health -longevity-mice-06398.html.

9. J. Donn et al., "Pharmaceuticals Lurking in U.S. Drinking Water," NBC News, March 10, 2008; nbcnews.com/id/23503485/ns/health-health_care/t /pharmaceuticals-lurking-us-drinking-water/#.XCaJzVxKi70.

10. Environmental Working Group, "Bottled Water Quality Investigation," October 15, 2008; ewg.org/research/bottled-water-quality-investigation /test-results-chemicals-bottled-water.

11. S. Lunder, "Pesticides + Poison Gasses = Cheap, Year-Round Strawberries," Environmental Working Group, April 10, 2018; ewg.org/foodnews /strawberries.php.

12. "Eat the Peach, Not the Pesticide," *Consumer Reports*, March 19, 2015; consumerreports.org/cro/health/natural-health/pesticides/index.htm.

13. S. Scutti, "You Can Cut Your Cancer Risk by Eating Organic, a New Study Says," CNN, October 22, 2018; cnn.com/2018/10/22/health/organic-food -cancer-study/index.html.

14. "Beef Feeding Research Studies Pasture Vs. Grain," *Science Daily*, April 7, 2005; sciencedaily.com/releases/2005/03/050329125520.htm.

15. H. D. Karsten et al., "Vitamins A, E and Fatty Acid Composition of the Eggs of Caged Hens and Pastured Hens," *Renewable Agriculture and Food Systems*, March 2010, 25(1): 45–54; cambridge.org/core/journals/renewable -agriculture-and-food-systems/article/vitamins-a-e-and-fatty-acid -composition-of-the-eggs-of-caged-hens-and-pastured-hens/552BA04E5A9E 3CD7E49E405B339ECA32.

16. A. Rock, "How Safe Is Your Ground Beef?" *Consumer Reports*, December 21, 2015; consumerreports.org/cro/food/how-safe-is-your-ground-beef.

17. A. MacMillan, "Exercise Makes You Younger at the Cellular Level," *Time*, May 15, 2017; time.com/4776345/exercise-aging-telomeres/.

18. R. D. Pollock, et al., "Properties of the Vastus Lateralis Muscle in Relation to Age and Physiological Function in Master Cyclists Aged 55 79 Years," *Aging Cell*, April 2018, 17(2): e12735; onlinelibrary.wiley.com/doi/full/10.1111 /acel.12735; N. A. Duggal et al., "Major Features of Immunosenescence, Including Thymic Atrophy, Are Ameliorated by High Levels of Physical Activity in Adulthood," *Aging Cell*, April 2018, 17(2): e12750; onlinelibrary.wiley .com/doi/full/10.1111/acel.12750; and "A Lifetime of Regular Exercise Slows Down Aging, Study Finds," *Science Daily*, March 8, 2018; sciencedaily.com /releases/2018/03/180308143123.htm.

19. K. A. Stokes et al., "The Time Course of the Human Growth Hormone Response to a 6 S and a 30 S Cycle Ergometer Sprint," *Journal of Sports Science*, June 2002, 20(6): 487–94; ncbi.nlm.nih.gov/pubmed/12137178.

20. "How Exercise—Interval Training in Particular—Helps Your Mitochondria Stave Off Old Age," *Science Daily*, March 7, 2017; sciencedaily.com /releases/2017/03/170307155214.htm.

21. N. Phillips, "Forget the Jog Slog and Fit in a Sprint for Maximum Weight Loss Results," *Sydney Morning Herald*, June 29, 2012; smh.com.au/lifestyle /forget-the-jog-slog-and-fit-in-a-sprint-for-maximum-weight-loss-results -20120628-215a4.html.

22. S. Melov et al., "Resistance Exercise Reverses Aging in Human

Skeletal Muscle," *PLoS ONE*, 2007, 2(5): e465; journals.plos.org/plosone/article /comments?id=10.1371/journal.pone.0000465; see also L. Kravitz, "Yes, Resistance Training Can Reverse the Aging Process," University of New Mexico; unm.edu/~lkravitz/Article%20folder/ageresistUNM.html.

23. "Lose Fat Faster Before Breakfast," *Science News*, January 24, 2013; science daily.com/releases/2013/01/130124091425.htm.

24. "Insufficient Sleep Could Be Adding to Your Waistline," University of Leeds, July 28, 2017; leeds.ac.uk/news/article/4079/insufficient_sleep_could _be_adding_to_your_waistline.

25. A. Gardner, "Too Little Sleep May Fuel Insulin Resistance," CNN, October 16, 2010; cnn.com/2012/10/15/health/sleep-insulin-resistance/index .html.

26. "The Effects of Sleep Deprivation," Johns Hopkins Medicine; hopkinsmedicine.org/health/healthy-sleep/health-risks/the-effects-of-sleep-deprivation.

27. "Blue Light Has a Dark Side," *Harvard Health Letter*, August 13, 2018; health .harvard.edu/staying-healthy/blue-light-has-a-dark-side.

28. T. L. Jacobs et al., "Self-Reported Mindfulness and Cortisol During a Shamatha Meditation Retreat," *Health Psychology*, October 2013, 32(10): 1104–09; ncbi.nlm.nih.gov/pubmed/23527522.

29. J. Marchant, "Mindfulness and Meditation Dampen Down Inflammation Genes," *New Scientist*, June 16, 2017; newscientist.com/article/2137595 -mindfulness-and-meditation-dampen-down-inflammation-genes/.

30. B. K. Hölzel et al., "Mindfulness Practice Leads to Increases in Regional Brain Gray Matter Density," *Psychiatry Research: Neuroimaging*, January 30, 2011, 191(1): 36–43; sciencedirect.com/science/article/pii/S092549271000288X.

31. F. Zeidan et al., "Mindfulness-Meditation-Based Pain Relief Is Not Mediated by Endogenous Opioids," *Journal of Neuroscience*, March 16, 2016, 36(11): 3391–97; ncbi.nlm.nih.gov/pmc/articles/PMC4792946/.

32. S. Lu, "Mindfulness Holds Promise for Treating Depression," *Monitor on Psychology*, American Psychological Association, March 2015; apa.org /monitor/2015/03/cover-mindfulness.aspx.

33. C. Tomiyama et al., "The Effect of Repetitive Mild Hyperthermia on Body Temperature, the Autonomic Nervous System, and Innate and Adaptive Immunity," *Biomedical Research*, 2015, 36(2): 135–42; jstage.jst.go.jp/article /biomedres/36/2/36_135/_pdf/-char/en.

34. M. E. Sears et al., "Arsenic, Cadmium, Lead, and Mercury in Sweat: A Systematic Review," *Journal of Environmental and Public Health*, February 22, 2012 (online); ncbi.nlm.nih.gov/pmc/articles/PMC3312275/.

35. S. J. Genuis et al., "Human Excretion of Bisphenol A: Blood, Urine, and Sweat

(BUS) Study," *Journal of Environmental and Public Health,* December 27, 2011; ncbi.nlm.nih.gov/pubmed/22253637.

36. A. MacMillan, "The Surprising Health Benefits of Saunas," *Time,* October 4, 2017; time.com/4967605/sauna-lower-blood-pressure/.

37. J. A. Laukkanen and T. Laukkanen, "Sauna Bathing and Systemic Inflammation," *European Journal of Epidemiology,* March 2018, 33(3); 351–53; ncbi.nlm.nih.gov/pubmed/29209938.

38. M. Krause et al., "Heat Shock Proteins and Heat Therapy for Type 2 Diabetes: Pros and Cons," *Current Opinion in Clinical Nutrition and Metabolic Care,* July 2015, 18(4): 374–80; ncbi.nlm.nih.gov/pubmed/26049635.

39. T. Laukkanen et al., "Sauna Bathing Is Inversely Associated with Dementia and Alzheimer's Disease in Middle-Aged Finnish Men," *Age and Ageing,* March 1, 2017, 46(2): 245–49; ncbi.nlm.nih.gov/pubmed/27932366.

40. B. A. Russell et al., "Study to Determine the Efficacy of Combination LED Light Therapy (633 nm and 830 nm) in Facial Skin Rejuvenation," *Journal of Cosmetic and Laser Therapy,* December 2005, 7(3–4): 196–200; ncbi.nlm.nih.gov/pubmed/16414908.

41. B. J. Park et al., "The Physiological Effects of Shinrin-Yoku (Taking in the Forest Atmosphere or Forest Bathing): Evidence from Field Experiments in 24 Forests Across Japan," *Environmental Health and Preventive Medicine,* January 2010, 15(1): 18–26; ncbi.nlm.nih.gov/pubmed/19568835.

42. Q. Li et al., "Forest Bathing Enhances Human Natural Killer Activity and Expression of Anti Cancer Proteins," *International Journal of Immunopathology and Pharmacology,* April–June 2007, 20(2 Supp 2): 3–8; ncbi.nlm.nih.gov/pubmed/17903349.

43. M. Gascon et al., "Outdoor Blue Spaces, Human Health and Well-Being: a Systematic Review of Quantitative Studies," *International Journal of Hygiene and Environmental Health,* November 2017, 220(8), 1207–21; ncbi.nlm.nih.gov/pubmed/28843736.

44. A. O'Connor, "The Claim: Exposure to Plants and Parks Can Boost Immunity," *New York Times,* July 5, 2010; nytimes.com/2010/07/06/health/06real.html.

45. G. Chevalier et al., "The Effects of Grounding (Earthing) on Bodyworkers' Pain and Overall Quality of Life: a Randomized Controlled Trial," *Explore,* October 11, 2018 (online); sciencedirect.com/science/article/pii/S1550830718302519?via%3Dihub.

46. "About Pets and People," Centers for Disease Control and Prevention; cdc.gov/healthypets/health-benefits/index.html.

47. Kelly Lambert, *Lifting Depression* (New York: Basic Books, 2001).

48. R. Walaszek, "Impact of Classic Massage on Blood Pressure in Patients with Clinically Diagnosed Hypertension," *Journal of Traditional Chinese Medicine*, August 2015, 35(4): 396–401; ncbi.nlm.nih.gov/pubmed/26427108.

49. A. MacSween et al., "A Randomized Crossover Trial Comparing Thai and Swedish Massage for Fatigue and Depleted Energy," *Journal of Bodywork and Movement Therapies*, July 2018, 22(3): 817–28; ncbi.nlm.nih.gov/pubmed/30100318.

50. H. Tang et al., "Treatment of Insomnia with Shujing Massage Therapy: a Randomized Controlled Trial," *Zhongguo Zhen Jiu*, August 2015, 35(8): 816–18; ncbi.nlm.nih.gov/pubmed/26571900.

51. S. Toprak Celenay et al., "A Comparison of the Effects of Exercises Plus Connective Tissue Massage to Exercises Alone in Women with Fibromyalgia Syndrome: a Randomized Controlled Trial," *Rheumatology International*, November 2017, 37(11): 1799–1806; ncbi.nlm.nih.gov/pubmed/28840379.

52. M. Hernandez-Reif et al., "Premenstrual Symptoms Are Relieved by Massage Therapy," *Journal of Psychosomatic Obstetrics and Gynecology*, April 2000, 21(1): 9–15; researchgate.net/publication/12412655_Premenstrual_symptoms_are_relieved_by_massage_therapy.

53. M. Grothaus, "Why Journaling Is Good for Your Health (And 8 Tips to Get Better)," *Fast Company*, January 29, 2015; fastcompany.com/3041487/8-tips-to-more-effective-journaling-for-health.

54. A. M. Seaman, "Acupuncture as Good as Counseling for Depression: Study," Reuters, September 24, 2013; reuters.com/article/us-acupuncture-depression-idUSBRE98N17420130924.

55. A. Firouzjaei, "Comparative Evaluation of the Therapeutic Effect of Metformin Monotherapy with Metformin and Acupuncture Combined Therapy on Weight Loss and Insulin Sensitivity in Diabetic Patients," *Nutrition & Diabetes*, May 2, 2016, 6(5): e209; ncbi.nlm.nih.gov/pmc/articles/PMC4895377/.

56. M. Narimani et al., "Effect of Acupressure on Pain Severity in Patients Undergoing Coronary Artery Graft: a Randomized Controlled Trial," *Anesthesiology and Pain Medicine*, October 20, 2018, 8(5): e82920; ncbi.nlm.nih.gov/pubmed/30538941.

57. N. T. T. Hmwe et al., "An Integrative Review of Acupressure Interventions for Older People: a Focus on Sleep Quality, Depression, Anxiety, and Agitation," *Internal Journal of Geriatric Psychiatry*, November 14, 2018; ncbi.nlm.nih.gov/pubmed/30430640.

Chapter 8

1. J. K. Tobacman, "Review of Harmful Gastrointestinal Effects of Carrageenan in Animal Experiments," *Environmental Health Perspectives*, October 2001,

109(10): 983–94; ncbi.nlm.nih.gov/pmc/articles/PMC1242073/pdf/ehp0109 -000983.pdf.

2. "Seaweed Suspect," VA Research Currents, February 2013; research.va.gov /currents/feb13/feb13-06.cfm.

3. Ibid.

Chapter 9

1. D. Ferriday et al., "Effects of Eating Rate on Satiety: a Role for Episodic Memory?," *Physiology & Behavior*, December 1, 2015, 152(Pt B): 389–96; ncbi .nlm.nih.gov/pubmed/26143189.

Chapter 10

1. M. Boschmann et al., "Water-Induced Thermogenesis," *Journal of Clinical Endocrinology & Metabolism*, December 1, 2003, 88(12): 6015–19; academic.oup .com/jcem/article/88/12/6015/2661518.

2. A. Madjd et al.,"Effects on Weight Loss in Adults of Replacing Diet Beverages with Water During a Hypoenergetic Diet: a Randomized, 24-Wk Clinical Trial," *American Journal of Clinical Nutrition*, December 2015, 102(6): 1305–12; academic.oup.com/ajcn/article/102/6/1305/4555169.

3. "Chronic Dehydration More Common Than You Think," CBS Miami, July 2, 2013; miami.cbslocal.com/2013/07/02/chronic-dehydration-more -common-than-you-think/.

Index

Also by **KELLYANN PETRUCCI**

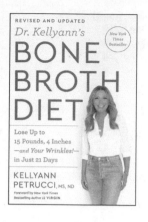

The book that started the bone broth movement. Now revised and updated.

Delicious recipes packed with essential nutrients for glowing health, firmer skin, and a healthier gut.

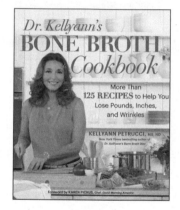

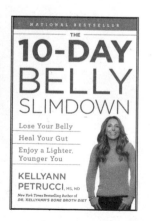

Heal your belly from the inside out and experience sustained weight loss.

RODALE.
BOOKS

Available wherever books are sold